Praise for the *New York Times* bestselling
The NEW Glucose Revolution Series

"The concept of the glycemic index has been distorted and bastardized by popular writers and diet gurus. Here, at last, is a book that explains what we know about the glycemic index and its importance in designing a diet for optimum health. Carbohydrates are not all bad. Read the good news about pasta and even—believe it or not—sugar!"
> —Andrew Weil, M.D., University of Arizona College of Medicine, author of *Spontaneous Healing* and *8 Weeks to Optimum Health,* on *The Glucose Revolution*

"The concept of glycemic index is key to understanding the effects of carbohydrate on human health. *The Low GI Handbook,* written by leading scientists, conveys this information clearly, thoroughly, and convincingly."
> —Walter Willett, Professor of Epidemiology and Nutrition, Harvard School of Public Health

"Jennie Brand-Miller and her research colleagues have done pioneering work, showing how the glycemic index can help you lose weight and improve your health. They are leading scientific authorities, and I often rely on their important findings in our research studies to help people reduce weight, control diabetes, tackle triglycerides, and return to health."
> —Neal Barnard, M.D., founder and president, Physicians for Responsible Medicine, and bestselling author

"Forget *SugarBusters*. Forget *The Zone*. If you want the real scoop on how carbohydrates and sugar affect your body, read this book by the world's leading researchers on the subject. It's the authoritative, last word on choosing foods to control your blood sugar."
> —Jean Carper, bestselling author of *Miracle Cures, Stop Aging Now!* and *Food: Your Miracle Medicine,* on *The Glucose Revolution*

"Clear, accessible, and authoritative information about the glycemic index. An exciting, new approach to preventing obesity, diabetes, and heart disease—written by internationally recognized experts in the field."
> —David Ludwig, M.D., Ph.D., director, Obesity Program, Children's Hospital, Boston, on *The New Glucose Revolution*

"Mounting evidence indicates that refined carbohydrates and high glycemic index foods are contributing to the escalating epidemics of obesity and type 2 diabetes worldwide. This dietary pattern also appears to increase the risk of heart disease and stroke. The skyrocketing proportion of calories from added sugars and refined carbohydrates in Westernized diets portends a future acceleration of these trends. *The Glucose Revolution* challenges traditional doctrines about optimal nutrition and the role of carbohydrates in health and disease. Brand-Miller and colleagues are to be congratulated for an eminently lucid and important book that explains the science behind the glycemic index and provides tools and strategies for modifying diet to incorporate this knowledge. I strongly recommend the book to both health professionals and the general public who could use this state-of-the-art information to improve health and well-being."

    —JoAnn E. Manson, M.D., Dr.P.H., professor of medicine,
    Harvard Medical School and codirector of Women's Health,
    Division of Preventive Medicine, Brigham and Women's
    Hospital

"Here is at last a book explaining the importance of taking into consideration the glycemic index values of foods for overall health, athletic performance, and in reducing the risk of heart disease and diabetes. The book clearly explains that there are different kinds of carbohydrates that work in different ways and why a universal recommendation to increase the carbohydrate content of your diet is plainly simple and scientifically inaccurate. Everyone should put the glycemic index approach into practice."

    —Artemis P. Simopoulos, M.D., senior author of *The Omega*
    Diet and *The Healing Diet* and president, The Center for
    Genetics, Nutrition and Health, Washington, D.C., on
    The Glucose Revolution

"*The Glucose Revolution* is nutrition science for the twenty-first century. Clearly written, it gives the scientific rationale for why all carbohydrates are not created equal. It is a practical guide for both professionals and patients. The food suggestions and recipes are exciting and tasty."

    —Richard N. Podell, M.D., M.P.H., clinical professor, Department of Family Medicine, UMDNJ-Robert Wood Johnson
    Medical School, and coauthor of *The G-Index Diet: The Missing*
    Link That Makes Permanent Weight Loss Possible

"The glycemic index is a useful tool which may have a broad spectrum of applications, from the maintenance of fuel supply during exercise to the control of blood glucose levels in diabetics. Low glycemic index foods may prove to have beneficial health effects for all of us in the long term. *The Glucose Revolution* is a user-friendly, easy-to-read overview of all that you need to know about the glycemic index. This book represents a balanced account of the importance of the glycemic index based on sound scientific evidence."

    —James Hill, Ph.D., director, Center for Human Nutrition,
    University of Colorado Health Sciences Center

"*The New Glucose Revolution* summarizes much of the recent development of dietary glycemic index and load in a highly readable format. The authors are able researchers and respected leaders in the nutrition field. Much that is discussed in this book draws directly from their years of experimental and observational research. The focus on dietary intervention and prevention strategies in everyday eating is an especially laudable feature of this book. I recommend this book most highly as an indispensable source of good nutrition."

    —Simin Liu, M.D., Sc.D., assistant professor, Department of
    Epidemiology, Harvard School of Public Health

"As a coach of elite amateur and professional athletes, I know how critical the glycemic index is to sports performance. *The New Glucose Revolution* provides the serious athlete with the basic tools necessary for getting the training table right."

    —Joe Friel, coach, author, consultant

Other titles in the New Glucose Revolution Series

We have put together this handy guide to help you make the right choice for further reading or for more recipes.

*The Low GI Handbook: The New Glucose Revolution Guide to the
Long-term Health Benefits of Low GI Eating*

COOKBOOKS

The Low GI Diet Cookbook: 100 Simple, Delicious Smart-Carb Recipes
The New Glucose Revolution Low GI Vegetarian Cookbook
The New Glucose Revolution Low GI Family Cookbook

SHOPPING AND EATING OUT

The New Glucose Revolution Shopper's Guide to GI Values 2010

DIABETES AND PREDIABETES

The New Glucose Revolution for Diabetes
The New Glucose Revolution Low GI Guide to Diabetes
What Makes My Blood Glucose Go Up . . . and Down?: 101 Frequently Asked Questions about Your Blood Glucose Level

WEIGHT LOSS

The Low GI Diet Revolution: The Definitive Science-Based Weight Loss Plan
The New Glucose Revolution Low GI Guide to Losing Weight

HEART HEALTH

*The New Glucose Revolution Low GI Guide to Your Heart
and the Metabolic Syndrome*

CELIAC DISEASE OR GLUTEN INTOLERANCE

The New Glucose Revolution Low GI Guide to Gluten-free Living

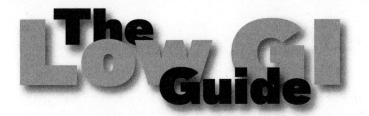

The Low GI Guide

to Living Well with

PCOS

Lose Weight, Boost Fertility and Gain Control over Polycystic Ovarian Syndrome with the Glycemic Index

Jennie Brand-Miller, Ph.D.
Nadir R. Farid, M.D.
Kate Marsh, Ph.D., R.D., C.D.E.

Recipes by
Chrissy Freer, Alison Roberts, Tracy Rutherford,
Philippa Sandall, and Diane Temple

Da Capo
LIFE
LONG

A Member of the Perseus Books Group

Recipes on pages 131, 132, 140, 144, 146, 148, 150, 152, 153 from *The New Glucose Revolution Low GI Vegetarian Cookbook*

Recipes by Chrissy Freer, Alison Roberts, Tracy Rutherford, Philippa Sandall, and Diane Temple

This is a completely revised edition of *The New Glucose Revolution Guide to Living Well with PCOS*, published in North America by Da Capo Press in 2004 and published in somewhat different form in Australia in 2004 under the title *The New Glucose Revolution Managing PCOS* by Hachette Livre Australia. This revised edition is published by arrangement with Hachette Livre Australia.

Set in ITC Legacy Serif by the Perseus Books Group

Cataloging-in-Publication Data is available from the Library of Congress.
ISBN 978-0-7382-1390-3

Published by Da Capo Press
A Member of the Perseus Books Group
www.dacapopress.com

Da Capo Press books are available at special discounts for bulk purchases in the U.S. by corporations, institutions, and other organizations. For more information, please contact the Special Markets Department at the Perseus Books Group, 2300 Chestnut Street, Suite 200, Philadelphia, PA, 19103, or call (800) 810-4145, extension 5000, or e-mail special.markets@perseusbooks.com.

10 9 8 7 6 5 4 3 2 1

Contents

Introduction

Why we wrote this book

CHANCES ARE YOU'VE PICKED UP THIS BOOK because you, or your doctor, suspect that you have PCOS—the popular shorthand for polycystic ovarian syndrome—and you want to find out more about it.

No doubt you've got plenty of questions and want some simple, straightforward answers. What exactly is PCOS? What are the signs and symptoms? How is the diagnosis confirmed? What causes it? Why *you*? And most importantly, what can you do about it? These are the types of questions we often get asked as professionals working daily with women with PCOS.

We wrote this book to try and give you some answers, and to give you the practical tools you need to help improve the underlying cause of PCOS: insulin resistance—a condition in which the body resists the actions of the hormone insulin.

What's more, we'll show you *how* you can improve your insulin sensitivity, step by step, with a delicious low-GI diet that's so effective, you'll want to stick to it for life. Not only will you lose weight in the first few months, you'll eat till you're satisfied and you'll never feel hungry. And none of your favorite foods are excluded entirely. Once you've lost weight, we do what other diet books don't—we give you a long-term eating plan to ensure you keep that weight off for life. And we explain how the GI fits in with other health messages about different types of fat and protein, showing you how easy it is to expand your healthy eating choices.

Diet won't be the only thing you change, of course. Exercise and medication are also important tools, but without key dietary changes, you'll be doing it the hard way. So, congratulate yourself, you've picked the right book to start managing your PCOS. As you read on you'll discover lots of real-life stories showing exactly how exercise, healthy low-GI eating, and the right medication can balance hormones, reduce insulin resistance, help beat the symptoms of PCOS, and, best of all, enable you to take charge.

In this revised version of our book, we have incorporated all the latest findings with respect to managing PCOS through lifestyle changes. We have also provided more details on exercise for women with PCOS and have included a range of new menus and recipes, including vegetarian and gluten-free options.

What's so different about the low-GI diet?

The low-GI Diet is a lifelong eating plan, not a calorie-restrictive diet. It's a groundbreaking way of eating based on what is known as the glycemic index (GI), which is the scientifically proven way of describing how carbohydrates in individual foods affect blood glucose levels. What you need to understand about the GI is that:

- Foods containing carbohydrates that break down quickly during digestion, releasing glucose quickly into the bloodstream, have a high GI.
- Foods containing carbohydrates that break down slowly, releasing glucose into the bloodstream gradually, have a low GI.

Low-GI foods are our key to achieving weight loss and blood glucose control. In turn, these will lead to more effective management of your PCOS symptoms. If you make the change and base your diet around healthy low-GI foods you will achieve lower insulin levels, making it easier for your body to burn fat and less likely that fat will be stored. Eating plenty of healthy low-GI foods will also:

- help lower your blood fats
- make you feel "full" and thus reduce appetite
- reduce your risk of developing diabetes
- improve your overall health

These aren't claims. These are facts that have been confirmed in numerous worldwide scientific studies.

In *The Low GI Guide to Living Well with PCOS* we show you how easy it is to include more of the right sort of low-GI carbohydrates in your diet every day and in every meal; which common foods have a low GI; and how you can make the GI work for you throughout the day with:

- practical hints for changing your eating habits
- quick and easy, healthy, low-GI, low-calorie recipes, meal ideas, and snacks

You are not alone

If you have PCOS, you are not alone. PCOS is thought to affect between 5 and 10 percent of women in developed nations. At the root of PCOS is insulin resistance. In the next chapter, we explain exactly what insulin resistance is. We will show you that there's plenty you can do about it, starting with diet and exercise.

And remember: a diet that is good for a woman who has PCOS is a diet that's good for everybody, every day, every meal. The signs of PCOS range from subtle symptoms, such as faint facial hair, to a "full house" syndrome—lack of periods, infertility, heavy body-hair growth, obstinate body fat, diabetes, and cardiovascular disease.

The symptoms of PCOS can occur at any age. Insulin resistance rises naturally at puberty, so PCOS can be seen in girls as young as ten or twelve years old. What's more, it does not suddenly disappear when the ovaries retire at menopause. Management of insulin resistance should continue beyond menopause as a supplement to other health-enhancing lifestyle measures.

It's vital to diagnose and treat women and girls as early as possible in order to prevent their PCOS from progressing to the "full-house" syndrome. The outdated view that early signs are "clinically insignificant"

Insulin Resistance

Insulin resistance is at the root of PCOS. We now know that more than half the population is insulin resistant—men and women, young and old. Insulin resistance is a chameleon that shows itself in many ways, differing from one person to another and between men and women. At one extreme, an individual may have only mildly abnormal blood tests. At the other, she (or he) may have a severe condition such as diabetes that impacts negatively on health, quality of life, and life expectancy.

and not worthy of proper management is simply not true. In fact, the sooner you (and your doctor) act, the better. As well as advice on medical management, diet and exercise, we also offer you tips on overcoming the stress and sleep problems that come hand in hand with PCOS. This is a total lifestyle plan for helping you manage your PCOS. It's your choice to adopt a program that ensures your present and future health. We have written this book to help you make that choice.

Knowledge is definitely power when it comes to your health. So, first up, we answer those pressing questions women ask about PCOS, its causes and medical management. In Chapter 2 we get down to detail on understanding the glycemic index, or GI for short, and the diet revolution we have been part of for over twenty years. A diet revolution that is now taking the whole world by storm. For the practical know-how to put it all into practice day by day, turn to Chapter 3 and check out the expert advice from a dietitian with more experience in managing PCOS than just about anyone else around. And finally we fill you up with delicious low-GI recipes specially devised by Alison Roberts and Tracy Rutherford, along with 16 new recipes for this new edition, that you will enjoy preparing time and again as you reap the benefits of healthy low-GI eating.

We believe understanding is very important if you are going to take charge and manage your PCOS, so we have included a glossary of technical terms at the back of the book as a quick reference. In the further reading section you will also find a list of organizations that will provide you with support and put you in contact with other women with PCOS, plus lots of Web sites and references you can follow up if you want to find out more.

> **"My experience so far has ensured a lifetime of lower GI eating for myself and my family."**
> *—Fiona*
>
> "I am currently pregnant with my third child. I was diagnosed with PCOS in 1998. Although my specialist at the time specialized in PCOS for her doctorate, I had no understanding of the link between insulin and my condition. I went on to have two rather large sons—10 pounds at 37 weeks and 10 pounds, 2 ounces at 35 weeks (yes, that is right!)—and gained a lot of weight during pregnancy. My second son also had blood glucose issues after birth, although I have never tested positive for gestational diabetes. In my journey to try and fall pregnant a third time I finally read a book I had owned for four years but never read—*The Low GI Guide to Living Well with PCOS*. What an eye opener! I can't believe I had not got around to reading it before. As my husband was also trying to lose weight at the time, I took the opportunity to switch to a low-GI diet. I have since become pregnant again and, despite not being rigid in my diet, have only gained a 'normal' amount of weight and the baby is measuring average for dates at five months. My experience so far has ensured a lifetime of lower GI eating for myself and my family (at least while I have some control over what goes in their mouths!)."
>
> *Update*: Fiona had baby number 3 in May—a very respectable 8 pounds, 7 ounces. "I know that is big for some but small for me! No blood glucose issues with the baby either," says Fiona.

1

Understanding PCOS

How can I tell if I have PCOS?

ONLY A DOCTOR CAN DIAGNOSE PCOS. But here's a list of the subtle symptoms of PCOS—not all of which need be present:

- delayed (or early) puberty
- irregular or no periods
- acne
- excess body or facial hair
- unexplained fatigue
- hypoglycemia (low blood glucose) after meals. The most common symptoms are light-headedness, sweating, sudden fatigue, and butterflies in the tummy
- excess weight around the waistline
- infertility
- mood swings
- hot flashes (heat intolerance and excess sweating) in young women
- sleep disorders, such as sleep apnea
- recurrent spontaneous miscarriages

- inappropriate lactation
- drop in blood pressure on standing up suddenly or with exercise
- acanthosis nigricans: rough, dark skin in the neck folds and armpits; a mark of severe insulin resistance from any cause

If you have one or more of these signs or symptoms, you should make an appointment with your doctor. They may refer you to an endocrinologist who specializes in PCOS.

A little history

Although polycystic ovaries were first described in France way back in 1844, it was two New York gynecologists, Irving F. Stein and Michael L. Leventhal, who diagnosed women with what we now consider to be severe PCOS and coined the term in 1935. The women that they described suffered from amenorrhea (no periods), severe hirsutism (unwanted hair), and polycystic ovaries (large ovaries with multiple cysts).

PCOS is more common than you'd expect

Up to 10 percent of women in industrialized countries have PCOS and the vast majority of them do not even suspect it. PCOS should be suspected in anyone with excess weight around the waist, excessive hair in the wrong places, acne, irregular periods, no periods, or problems getting pregnant. Young women who require insulin to control their diabetes are also at risk of developing PCOS.

Symptoms of PCOS usually first appear around menarche (the first period), but can occur anytime during a woman's reproductive life. Subtle symptoms such as hot flushes (long before menopause), otherwise unexplained weight gain, mood swings, hirsutism, and "hypoglycemia" (low blood glucose) after meals may be suggestive of PCOS. Despite its name, PCOS involves the whole body and not just the ovaries. This is why it is so important to identify girls who are at risk *before* they reach puberty. If PCOS can be treated early, there are lifelong health benefits.

The ovary is a sensitive beacon for insulin resistance and thus allows early recognition of a metabolic problem. Having PCOS in-

I have PCOS and know it is genetic. Is there any way I can prevent my baby girl from getting it?

This question is a difficult one to answer. There are no specific guidelines for preventing PCOS. We do know that it is genetic and therefore the best thing to do is to eat a healthy diet and be active as a family and hopefully she will adopt these good habits as she grows! Current research suggests that diets low in saturated fat and high in fiber are associated with a lower risk of diabetes as are diets with more whole grains and a lower GI. Since the underlying problem in both type 2 diabetes and PCOS (in most cases) is insulin resistance, these findings are also relevant to women with PCOS. We also know that exercising regularly protects against diabetes and improves insulin sensitivity. And of course, a combination of healthy eating and regular physical activity helps with weight management, which also helps with insulin sensitivity. Ensuring your daughter has a healthy rate of weight gain as she grows (not too much or too little) may also help in reducing her risks of health problems, including PCOS.

So, the best advice we can give right now is for you to encourage your daughter as she grows to eat a good variety of fruits, vegetables and whole grains, lean protein foods and dairy products (low fat varieties are not recommended for children under 2 years of age) or alternatives. Highly processed carbohydrate foods and those high in saturated fat and sugar with a poor nutritional value (e.g., cookies, pastries, chips, candy and soft drinks) are best kept for occasional treats rather than everyday choices. If you need some more specific advice, make an appointment to talk with a Registered Dietitian (RD) who has experience in PCOS to help you developing a healthy eating plan for her.

creases the likelihood that further medical problems will develop over time. These include: type 2 diabetes, heart disease, hypertension, fatty liver, and cancer of the uterus. We also know that serious sleep disorders and depression are much more common in women with PCOS. Alarmingly, women with PCOS who do get pregnant stand a 40 percent chance of spontaneous miscarriage in the first three months of pregnancy. There is also an increased risk of gestational diabetes, multiple pregnancies, and in later pregnancy, preeclampsia

The Normal Female Cycle

To understand PCOS you need to understand the normal menstrual cycle.

The hypothalamus in the brain signals the pituitary gland to secrete FSH (follicle-stimulating hormone) and LH (luteinizing hormone). In the first half of the cycle, these pulses are infrequent and FSH is secreted preferentially, allowing a crop of follicles to grow inside the ovaries. This phase is therefore called the "follicular" phase. The follicles secrete estrogen and acquire receptors for LH. As estrogen levels rise, the hypothalamus pulses more and more frequently. Estrogen stimulates the growth of the breasts and of the lining of the uterus. Most of the follicles degenerate in the next few days and only one is mysteriously selected. This dominant follicle (the "egg") matures over the next few days, and just before ovulation—when the dominant follicle is expelled from the ovary—estrogen levels peak.

After ovulation, the dominant ruptured follicle becomes the corpus luteum. This little body secretes progesterone, the hormone that promotes the growth of blood vessels of the uterine lining in preparation of the implanting of a fertilized egg. This phase is called the luteal phase. If the egg is not fertilized, estrogen and progesterone levels fall, and the uterine lining is shed and menstruation occurs. At the time of puberty when girls have reached a critical muscle-to-fat ratio, the hypothalamus gives the GO signal for the start of menstruation. Excessive weight loss, exercise, or stress can negate that signal.

At the peak years of reproductive life most women have a regular 28-day cycle, plus or minus 2–3 days. The first day of the menstrual period is day 1. Ovulation usually occurs on day 14 to 15, but can occur anywhere from day 9 to 17 due to variability in the length of the follicular phase of the cycle. Around menarche and menopause, the cycles are irregular and often not associated with ovulation.

(a serious complication of late pregnancy that requires immediate medical attention). When a thorough medical check was carried out after delivery, a high percentage of women with gestational diabetes were found to have PCOS. Although direct evidence is not available, some doctors even suspect that PCOS will also turn out to be a risk factor for Alzheimer's disease.

Given the fact that it afflicts up to 10 percent of women of reproductive age, PCOS should be considered a health hazard for all women. Indeed, one wonders if it should be called a disease at all—PCOS is more than just a personal problem, because it affects so many women. It needs to be seen as a public health issue that deserves community support.

Doctors have to suspect it to diagnose it

The sooner you have a definite diagnosis of PCOS the better. That's because intervention and treatment will be more effective if "the full house" of symptoms has not yet set in. This requires a high level of suspicion on the part of your doctor. Here are the test results that should alert your doctor:

- A blood test showing that key hormones are abnormally high or low: testosterone that is too high, sex hormone binding globulin (SHBG) that is too low, and high levels of luteinizing hormone (LH) while follicle stimulating hormone (FSH) levels are normal.
- An ultrasound examination showing "bulky" ovaries with cysts. In thin women, ultrasound through the abdominal wall will allow good views of the uterus and ovaries, but for those who are overweight, internal ultrasound examination is often necessary.

It's important to stress that the symptoms, blood test results, and ultrasound findings need to be interpreted by a medical practitioner with experience in PCOS. Some women do not show the "classic" signs at all.

Some doctors make a distinction between polycystic ovarian *syndrome* (PCOS) and polycystic ovarian *disease* (PCOD). You may have heard both terms used. Both PCOS and PCOD are underpinned by the same metabolic problem—insulin resistance. They have to be treated in much the same way. For simplicity, throughout this book, we use the term PCOS to refer to both.

The insulin resistance link

Insulin resistance is a condition in which the body "resists" the normal actions of the hormone insulin; that is, the body's response to insulin is defective. To overcome this resistance, the body secretes more insulin than normal. The vast majority of women with PCOS have severe insulin resistance and therefore very high insulin levels.

Being overweight or obese increases the degree of insulin resistance, but you can be very lean and still have PCOS. You could also have PCOS as a result of an unusual inherited or acquired disease of the adrenal glands—it's pretty rare, but it should be considered by your doctor as part of the medical investigations as it requires specific treatment for the primary underlying condition.

My mom recommended that I see the doctor because I was trying to get pregnant (I had been married for nine months) but wasn't having much success. My periods were regular but they were longer than usual. I also had dark hairs growing up the naval line as well as on the inside of my upper thighs below the bikini-line. Because the hair growth was of recent onset, he immediately suspected PCOS, and sent me off for an ultrasound later the same afternoon. The ultrasound confirmed that both ovaries, but more so the right, were enlarged and contained multiple cysts.

I had some blood tests too which were suggestive of PCOS. He prescribed a healthy low-GI diet, exercise, and metformin. A few weeks later I went on a dream vacation to the Caribbean for two weeks, and on my return I was delighted to discover that I was pregnant! I have continued with the healthy low-GI diet and exercise program and I plan to stick to it for life.
    Louise, 27

What exactly is insulin resistance?

Whenever we eat, whatever the nature of the food, glucose and insulin levels in the blood rise and fall over the next couple of hours. Both carbohydrates and proteins in our food stimulate the secretion of insulin—it is essential for life. Insulin drives the transport of glucose (from digested carbohydrate) and amino acids (the building blocks of protein) into our cells, as well as the storage of glucose in the liver and our muscles.

Insulin can also suppress the use of fat as a source of fuel and the capacity of the liver to make new glucose molecules—neither of which is needed during the first hour or two after a meal. Think of insulin as a facilitator of "energy storage."

Beyond these roles in metabolism, insulin is important for growth before and after birth, and it's absolutely essential for the optimal functioning of many other hormones and enzymes. We are also beginning to learn about the role insulin plays in brain function, and thus behavior. While insulin has many functions in our bodies, carbohydrate metabolism is the only one that is affected by insulin resistance.

Like a lock and key mechanism, most body cells have special "receptors" for insulin. Once the lock is engaged—insulin attaches itself to the receptor—the gates open, allowing glucose to flow into the cell. The higher the concentration of insulin receptors, the more insulin sensitive you are.

If the number of insulin receptors is lower than normal or they are compromised in some way, then the cells are said to be "insulin resistant." The pancreas, the organ that secretes insulin, responds to this situation by secreting more insulin in an effort to overcome the block and achieve normal transport of glucose. One of the hallmarks of insulin resistance is therefore an inappropriately high level of insulin in the blood, both before and after meals.

Unfortunately, in many people, the pancreas has a limited capacity to secrete large amounts of insulin. It's only a matter of time before the cells burn out and they can't supply enough insulin to meet demand and the person develops prediabetes or the full-blown diabetic state.

How does excess insulin cause PCOS?

Great progress has been made in understanding the links between excess insulin and PCOS. Insulin stimulates the growth and multiplication of cells in the ovary, in particular those that make up the bulk of the ovary in which the eggs are embedded. Insulin resistance leads to a vicious cycle of hormonal imbalances that create the symptoms of PCOS.

I was diagnosed with PCOS about 20 years ago with most of the standard symptoms. My doctor did a glucose tolerance test, which came out to be normal. Why am I not showing any signs of insulin resistance, if PCOS is supposed to be caused by it?

Insulin resistance is the most common cause, and 70–80 percent of women with PCOS have insulin resistance. But a glucose tolerance test doesn't pick up insulin resistance; rather, it picks up the inability of the pancreas to deal with insulin resistance. If your pancreas has lots of "puff," your glucose tolerance will remain normal, perhaps all your life. Only a fraction of people with insulin resistance go on to develop impaired glucose tolerance. Nonetheless, high insulin levels can cause other problems downstream, and the ovaries are particularly sensitive. Any woman with diagnosed PCOS also needs to have the actual cause of the problem pinpointed so she gets the right treatment for her and thus the best outcomes. Some of the other causes are anorexia, bulimia, stress, excessive exercise, high blood levels of prolactin and tumors of the adrenal glands, ovaries, or pituitary gland. And for some women the cause is unknown.

The receptors for insulin in the ovary are different from those in other tissues, in that when blood insulin levels are high, the ovary does not turn down insulin receptor numbers or reduce their activity. Therefore, the action of insulin continues unabated in ovarian tissues. The cells grow and multiply, as well as increasing their metabolic activity. The result is excessive production of both male (testosterone) as well as female (estrogen) sex hormones. When the body is functioning healthily, men and women produce both sorts of hormones, although in vastly different proportions.

Insulin resistance leads to a vicious cycle of hormonal imbalances that create the symptoms of PCOS.

Normally, the ovary makes testosterone and then converts it to estrogen. However, excessive stimulation of the ovary overwhelms its capacity to fully undertake this conversion, with the result that excess testosterone spills over into the blood. The uncharacteristically high testosterone levels in the blood then bring about "male" characteristics in women, such as hirsutism and weight gain.

Excess insulin and sex hormones also work together to stimulate one of the areas in the brain called the hypothalamus, making it more sensitive. It "pulses" more frequently than normal, inducing the gland underneath—called the pituitary—to secrete more luteinizing hormone (LH for short). LH stimulates the ovary's hormone production even more—and a vicious cycle is up and running. Breaking that cycle is the key to managing PCOS successfully.

Excess insulin has even more consequences. It stimulates the conversion of weak male and female hormones to the more potent forms—estrogen and testosterone. And, finally, it reduces the level of the protein that binds testosterone in the blood. In this way, the active form of the hormone is made "more available" to the tissues.

Testosterone is called an anabolic hormone because it is involved in building up new tissues, especially muscles. This muscle-building potential is the main reason men have more muscle mass than women. It's also why unscrupulous athletes use it to enhance their performance. In women with PCOS, however, excess testosterone and other male hormones contribute to excessive weight gain and "masculinization."

It is this complicated interplay between insulin resistance, ovarian hormones, and increased pituitary stimulation of the ovaries that accounts for all the signs and hormonal features of PCOS.

How insulin causes excess body fat

Fat cells and their precursor cells in different parts of the human body are not all the same. Those around the midriff and inside the tummy are particularly sensitive to the effects of insulin compared with those in the rest of the body.

One of insulin's most powerful actions is to inhibit the release of fat from fat stores, making it difficult to call on abdominal fat as a source of fuel. In this way, midriff fat gradually accumulates around the waist, a sign that is typical of women and girls with PCOS. In fact, it is one of the most obvious and typical signs of insulin resistance in both women and men.

Can you inherit insulin resistance?

We know that insulin resistance is more common in some groups of people than others. For example, Asian people have been found to be more insulin resistant than people of Caucasian origin. And American Indians, Australian Aboriginals, and Pacific Islanders are more insulin resistant than most.

Not surprisingly, PCOS also runs in families and often there is a family history of type 2 diabetes too. Modern genetic analyses point the finger at several genes that suggest a predisposition to PCOS, but one of them in isolation is not sufficient to cause the disease. Many of the genes identified are involved in the action of insulin and in the production or metabolism of the sex hormones. So, to some extent you can blame your genes—and your parents!

Environmental factors and lack of physical exercise are also important. We know that weight gain can trigger insulin resistance and PCOS, as can steroid medication.

"PCOS" in Men

Some studies have shown the "trait" associated with PCOS in female members of a family also appeared to be passed on to some of the men in that family. Men are as liable to insulin resistance as women, but not having ovaries, the signs of the disease are different. Frontal baldness and, to a lesser measure, excessive body-hair growth, was once thought to indicate insulin resistance in male relatives; more recent studies have demonstrated that these factors are not reliable indicators of "PCOS in men." Rather it manifests itself as central obesity, carbohydrate craving, fatigue, sleep disorders, dyslipidemia, and fatty liver. Also, raised serum androstenedione has been found to be a telltale sign for affected male relatives. A recent study found that 42 percent of fathers and 22 percent of brothers of women with PCOS had the metabolic syndrome, compared to 32 percent and 9 percent of the general population. Another study found that brothers of women with PCOS had abnormal blood fats and insulin resistance, similar to their sisters.

We are less sure about the links between PCOS and stress or the use of contraceptives.

If you were born small—with a birth weight under 5½ pounds—you are more likely to be insulin resistant. Baby girls with low birth weight who then put on weight quickly within the first year or two of life are especially likely to develop PCOS at the time of their first period.

 PCOS also runs in families and often there is a family history of type 2 diabetes.

Why is insulin resistance so common?

Many of the women with PCOS that we meet wonder why something so seemingly undesirable would be so common and have a genetic basis. One popular theory that endeavors to explain the prevalence of insulin resistance is called the "thrifty genotype" hypothesis. According to this theory, our ancestors endured cycles of food scarcity and food abundance. Those individuals with a degree of insulin resistance had an advantage because their high insulin levels suppressed the use of fat as a fuel source, leading to greater body fat accumulation during periods of abundance. Then, when food was scarce, they could draw on those fat reserves. This survival advantage meant the genes for insulin resistance (i.e., the "thrifty" genes) spread throughout human populations.

An alternative theory, called the "carnivore connection" is gaining ground. According to this theory, genes for insulin resistance were particularly advantageous during the Ice Ages that characterized the last two million years of human evolution. When the planet was colder and drier, and plant growth was limited, human diets are thought to have become increasingly carnivorous—dependent on the large herds of animals that thrived on the steppes of Europe and the grasslands of Africa. Such diets are low in carbohydrates. Hence a metabolism that spared blood glucose for essential purposes, redirecting it away from muscles, would have had survival and reproductive advantages. The large human brain and the fetus are both exclusively dependent on glucose as a source of fuel—they cannot use fat. On this diet, the genes for insulin resistance may have become more and more common.

Whatever the reason—food scarcity in general, or just carbohydrates in short supply—it's clear that the genes for insulin resistance are no longer an advantage. In developed nations, food is too plentiful and our lifestyles too sedentary, and those previously advantageous metabolic attributes have come to prey upon our health. We have made our lifestyles just too easy for our own good.

Insulin resistance is now regarded as the underlying basis for all the diseases of affluence: obesity, prediabetes, type 2 diabetes, abnormal cholesterol levels, high blood pressure, coronary artery disease, fatty liver, preeclampsia, and PCOS. Who gets them? Disease is determined by your gender, diet, lifestyle, and how overweight you are—together with all those other genes you inherited from your mom and dad.

PCOS is a risk factor for further medical complications

Reducing your insulin resistance is vital, not only for tackling the symptoms of PCOS but also to minimize the complications that often follow insulin resistance. We want to emphasize that some of these risks are worst-case scenarios and can be prevented by the type of treatment and sensible lifestyle changes recommended in this book.

- the insulin resistance/metabolic syndrome
- type 2 diabetes
- coronary artery disease
- stroke
- early miscarriages
- multiple pregnancies
- preeclampsia
- uterine cancer
- depression
- Alzheimer's disease

I was referred to the endocrinologist because I often had dizzy spells and my doctor found one of two fasting blood glucose levels were a bit low. I went with my mom, Diane, because I'm shy and hate seeing doctors. The endocrinologist asked lots of questions and made me realize that I often felt light-headed, faint, and sweaty about two hours after some meals. He also pointed out that I was slightly overweight and had mild excess body hair growth. Although my blood pressure was normal, it showed a significant drop when he measured it as I was standing and that's when I felt faint. He found that I was insulin resistant and arranged for an ultrasound that day that showed that I had large polycystic ovaries. That's when he prescribed metformin plus a healthy low-GI diet with lots of vegetables and regular aerobic exercise (which I hate!).

Ruth, 18

Signs of the insulin resistance syndrome

Doctors can pinpoint the metabolic characteristics of anyone with *severe* insulin resistance. These days it's called the "metabolic syndrome" but it also goes by the name of "Syndrome X." If you have this syndrome, you won't necessarily show every characteristic listed below, but you will have at least two or three of them:

- a large waist circumference (also known as central obesity)
- high blood glucose (in the fasting state before breakfast or after meals)
- high blood pressure
- high blood triglyceride ("trigs")
- high levels of small, dense cholesterol
- low levels of HDL (the good cholesterol)
- fatty liver (nonalcoholic steatohepatitis or NASH)
- PCOS

My daughter Ruth was having dizzy spells, so I went to the doctor with her and that's when I learned all about insulin resistance and the fact that it runs in families. So I made an appointment to see the endocrinologist immediately. I am postmenopausal and a survivor of large bowel cancer. I am also a little overweight (the endocrinologist called it "centrally obese"). I have high blood pressure too. After examining me and sending me off for all kinds of tests, the doctor realized that I had all the signs of the metabolic syndrome including high cholesterol, low "good cholesterol," and high triglycerides, and high blood glucose two hours after a glucose drink. My heart tracing showed evidence of an old heart attack. He put me on metformin, a healthy low-GI diet, blood pressure tablets, and medications to lower my blood fats. And, of course, an exercise program.

Diane, 48

Left undiagnosed and untreated, a person with the metabolic syndrome will often go on to develop other more serious medical problems (see list on page 12).

Effective medical management of PCOS

The vast majority of women with PCOS are profoundly insulin resistant even if they are not overweight. Managing their PCOS requires an integrated program of lifestyle change and medication to achieve the treatment goals: weight loss if necessary, normalizing blood hormone levels, control of acne, resumption of ovulation, and regular periods.

The cornerstone of managing PCOS is lifestyle modification with a healthy low-GI diet and exercise. These changes need to be initiated right from the start, even before the use of insulin-sensitizing drugs.

It's also important to keep in mind that your treatment should be tailored to deal with your symptoms and, to some extent, your priorities. That might be regular periods, a much-wanted pregnancy, or simply a reduction in body hair.

Until recently, the most popular medical approach of treating PCOS was to "suppress ovarian function and replace estrogen" with an oral contraceptive pill. While this is effective, it does nothing to address the basic problem of insulin resistance, the underlying cause of PCOS. Moreover, because estrogen is one of the two components in the pill, long-term use carries the same risk as that for estrogen alone, including the risk of breast cancer.

In recent years, and with a better understanding of the metabolic basis of PCOS, the emphasis has shifted. Many doctors now direct their efforts to managing insulin resistance in PCOS with an integrated program of low-GI diet, regular aerobic exercises, and insulin-sensitizing drugs such as metformin.

The optimal dose of metformin is usually 500 milligrams three times a day with meals (there is also a newer slow release version called metformin XR which may be taken once per day, usually before bed) and can help with weight loss, normalization of hormonal levels (testosterone, LH, and insulin), resumption of regular periods, ovulation, and pregnancy. Research also suggests that metformin may help to prevent diabetes in those at risk. But the key to success is early diagnosis and treatment combined with a low-GI diet and exercise.

For women who become pregnant, research to date shows that it may be a good idea to continue metformin throughout pregnancy, particulary in the first twelve weeks, to prevent the otherwise higher likelihood of miscarriage and to reduce the risk of developing gestational diabetes. Metformin does not appear to harm the fetus, although it is currently not an approved medication for use during pregnancy—this may change soon as the results of longer-term studies become available.

In due course, newer insulin sensitizers that are more potent than metformin may become useful in the management of PCOS, either alone or in combination with metformin.

A new class of drugs called glitazones is being used successfully in the treatment of type 2 diabetes and the metabolic syndrome. These drugs work by sensitizing tissues to insulin and may be used in combination with metformin in women with PCOS. These medications should not, however, be used in those who wish to become pregnant.

Combinations of metformin and drugs that block the effect of testosterone on the body (e.g., spiranolactone or finasteride) have also been used in women with severe hirsutism. But, again, these drugs must be avoided for women wanting to become pregnant.

It was about eighteen months ago, at the age of 28, when I was diagnosed with PCOS. I'd been overweight for most of my twenties and had a history of irregular periods (not to mention a family history of diabetes). It

Metformin

Metformin, more commonly known as Glucophage, has been around for a long time. In fact, it has been used to treat people with type 2 diabetes for over fifty years. It has recently gained greater respect because we now know that it also helps prevent the long-term complications of diabetes, such as eye and coronary artery diseases.

Metformin works by reducing glucose production by the liver and increasing the uptake of glucose by the body (i.e., it increases insulin sensitivity). This is why it's so useful in treating women with PCOS. In fact, even before a woman with PCOS has achieved any significant weight loss, metformin can be effective in improving her other symptoms.

There are some side effects, however, including a metallic taste in the mouth, excess gas, and soft stools that may graduate to diarrhea. For most people, these are mild and disappear within a few weeks. However, to keep any possible side effects and discomfort to a minimum, doctors usually introduce metformin gradually over a period of three to four weeks, starting with a 500 milligram tablet after dinner for ten days. If this causes no major problems, then another 500 milligram tablet is introduced after breakfast and in another ten days another tablet is taken after lunch. Some women prefer to take their medication only twice a day and use 850 milligram tablets twice a day. The optimal dose is around 1500–1700 milligrams per day.

Metformin may interfere with the absorption of vitamin B_{12}. Hence it is important to have regular full blood counts to measure blood levels of B_{12}. If you have kidney or liver failure or serious circulatory problems, you should not take metformin at all. It is also important to avoid or limit alcohol while taking this medication.

It should be noted that in most countries no drug other than the contraceptive pill is licensed for the treatment of PCOS. Even metformin is not yet approved for this purpose.

had been six months since my last period and I knew I wasn't pregnant, so I had my doctor run some tests. At my next appointment she broke the news. It was Polycystic Ovary Syndrome in combination with Insulin Resistance. It was a real wake-up call. My father is a type 2 diabetic and I was heading in the same direction. The doctor's suggestion was a drug called Metformin to help with my weight and regulate my periods, the same medication my father was on for diabetes. To me, the concept of being on daily medication for the rest of my life, just to combat my symptoms, was unacceptable. So I began to educate myself on my condition and other alternatives to medication. I learned about the concept of "Low GI" and the importance of regular exercise in maintaining a healthy lifestyle. Then I set about changing my life by incorporating both, and, surprisingly, it wasn't that hard to do. I was already eating mostly the right foods, just in the wrong way, and the GI Diet taught me to balance it out. Now, three weeks away from my thirtieth birthday, I can honestly say I am the happiest I've ever been. I exercise most days, eat a healthy "Low GI" diet, and have a normal regular menstrual cycle. Not to mention I've lost nearly thirty pounds! My symptoms have disappeared and I'm medication free, all thanks to a little education and the GI Revolution.

Karen, 30

A much-wanted pregnancy

This book is primarily concerned with helping you to manage your PCOS symptoms on a daily basis.

I'm 29 and have PCOS. I was diagnosed in my early teens. My symptoms are irregular periods, infertility, and excess of testosterone levels (hormone imbalance). I didn't find out until this year that the main underlying problem was my insulin level. I did lots of research on my own about PCOS and if there was a way to reverse my condition because I wanted to start a family, and I found that being on a low-GI diet was the ticket. I'm not overweight (that can be another side effect of having PCOS), but after only three months of being on a low-GI diet, I lost ten pounds and my cycles became regular. Then the shock of my life came when I found out that I was pregnant—after all these years of doctors telling me that getting pregnant would be a great challenge or that it won't happen at all! And all because I stayed committed to a low-GI diet so that my insulin levels wouldn't rise too high. I've finally learned that we can reverse our health conditions once we have the knowledge of what the "trigger" is, and I believe in nature's way of doing this. Knowledge is power and I'm staying on the low-GI diet for as long as I can because I know I've seen the great results for myself.

I finally got pregnant!
Stephanie, 29

Unfortunately, there is not enough space here to have an in-depth look at assisted ovulation and pregnancy in women with PCOS. The measures recommended in this book: a low-GI diet, regular exercise, and metformin treatment will maximize the likelihood of regular ovulation, and eventually pregnancy. If ovulation is not achieved in four to six months of metformin treatment, other medical intervention should be considered. Many IVF programs pre-treat women—even those *without* PCOS—with metformin because it increases the chances of successful embryo implantation.

I consulted my family doctor because I just couldn't get pregnant despite being off the pill for over nine months. I certainly wasn't overweight, although I was a bit tubbier around the tummy than I liked and my periods had been pretty irregular for the last six months. My doctor suspected PCOS and sent me to have an ultrasound. That showed that both my ovaries were enlarged and had multiple cysts. He prescribed metformin, gave me a program of aerobic exercises, and referred me to a dietitian to learn all about healthy low-GI eating. I found the diet really easy to follow and at the same time built up the dose of metformin he had prescribed to a full dose with every meal. It seems amazing now, but just two months after I started this program I noticed that my tummy was flattening out. Best of all my periods were now regular and I was ovulating. The next month I missed my period. I was pregnant!
Claire, 26

Skin and hair

Acne and an oily complexion, usually appearing around the time of puberty, may be the very first signs of PCOS. Hard-to-treat acne and acne that appears later in life can also signal the possibility of PCOS. Acne associated with PCOS will respond to metformin and lifestyle changes, although in some cases the addition of antibiotics or andro-gen blockers may be necessary.

With treatment, excessive facial and body-hair growth will slow down. Hair will become finer as blood levels of the male sex hor-mones fall. The slow nature of hair growth, however, means that the benefits of any treatment will involve a wait of five to six months. In addition, many people with PCOS are still not satisfied with the level of excess body-hair growth despite metformin treatment, and their quality of life is affected. In these cases, testosterone blockers or drugs that influence testosterone metabolism are sometimes pre-scribed (e.g., flutamide). Recent studies show that it can be used at a fraction of the traditional dose. Unfortunately, this medication is not without side effects, and liver function tests must be carried out peri-odically and the drug discontinued if pregnancy is contemplated.

The contraceptive pill is effective in reducing excessive body hair too, but using it over a long-term period has been questioned. The water pill, spiranolactone, is less effective, although it has been used for many years at high doses for this purpose. It may be necessary to supplement the medical treatment of excess facial and body hair with those tried-and-true traditional methods for hair removal such as depilatory creams, electrolysis, flashlamps, intense pulsed light, and laser hair removal. Electrolysis and laser therapy, in particular, often lead to a dramatic improvement in quality of life. The cream "Vaniqa" when used alongside traditional methods has been found to be effective by most users.

Unfortunately, there are many products and procedures, includ-ing those for "permanent hair removal," that do not stand up to the claims of the manufacturers. An excellent guide to appropriate prod-ucts is: www.hairfacts.com.

The longer term

The longer your insulin resistance remains untreated the more likely you are to develop the metabolic syndrome, type 2 diabetes, or car-diovascular disease. Once treatment commences many doctors be-lieve that it's important for women with PCOS to continue medical management longer term and certainly beyond menopause. Lifestyle modification, including a healthy low-GI diet, exercise, and possibly pharmacological treatment, might therefore be lifelong. That makes it all the more critical that the diet and lifestyle you adopt is one you can stick to long term. Anything else will result in the "rhythm method of girth control"—cycles of weight loss and weight gain that could do more harm than good, not just to your health but to your sense of self-esteem.

This section of the book should have answered all your pressing questions about the causes of PCOS and its medical management. Now it's time to talk in detail about dietary management. In the next chapter we tell you all about the GI, the diet revolution that is taking the whole world by storm.

2

All about Carbohydrates and the GI of Foods

IN THIS CHAPTER we'll explain the whys and wherefores of making the change to a healthy diet that includes low-GI carbohydrates and how this will help you beat the symptoms of PCOS. Women with PCOS or diabetes have often told us that understanding the science behind the insulin connection made it logical and easy to make the change to a healthy low-GI diet.

As we showed in the previous chapter, insulin resistance is at the root of PCOS. But, you may well ask, what does this actually do to you? Well, it basically means that your body has a hard time bringing blood glucose levels down after you've eaten—no matter whether it's breakfast, lunch, or dinner, or just an in-between snack.

This is where low-GI diet comes in. It's a revolution so far-reaching that it will change the way you eat, the way you cook—even the way you think about food. The GI (glycemic index) is the scientifically proven way of describing how carbohydrates in individual foods actually affect our blood glucose levels.

The fact is, the GI, which started out as a dietary tool to help people with diabetes choose the right foods to control blood glucose, has become the way of eating that everyone's talking about today—and one of few nutritional programs with sound scientific research to support it.

Back to basics

A low-GI lifestyle makes a key contribution to helping you beat PCOS symptoms because it focuses on carbohydrates—their quantity *and* quality, and their overall effect on your blood glucose. Controlling your blood glucose levels is the first step to increasing your insulin sensitivity.

With so much coverage of carbohydrates ongoing in the media, it's easy to get confused between low-carb and high-carb diets. Carbohydrates are nature's primary fuel, and a very important food for health and energy. In our low-GI diet books we focus not just on carbohydrate quantity—though it is important as you will see later in this chapter—but also on carbohydrate *quality*, or, more specifically, the nature of the carbohydrate and its overall effect on our blood glucose. You can find out the quantity of carbohydrate in foods pretty easily—it's usually on the packaging, or you can look in one of those little food-counter books. Making a decision about carbohydrate quality, however, can be guesswork. The old complex-versus-simple-carbohydrate approach doesn't tell the true story.

What will tell you something about carbohydrate "quality" is a food's GI. We discuss the GI in more detail later in this chapter, for now all you need to know is that the GI is just a number (actually it's a ranking) that reflects the glycemic potential of carbohydrates: their ability to raise your blood glucose levels. Depending on the source of the carbohydrates (i.e., the actual food as prepared and eaten), they can raise blood glucose levels quite a lot, or just a little.

Healthy low-GI foods are the key to achieving weight loss, blood glucose control, and lifelong health. If you make the change and base your diet around eating balanced low-GI meals, you will achieve lower insulin levels, making it easier for your body to burn fat and less likely that fat will be stored in all those places you don't want it. Unlike a low-carbohydrate diet, eating the low-GI way is healthy, balanced, and safe for children and adults alike. Not only that, it helps you expand your healthy eating choices, lose weight, feel fuller, and manage many of your PCOS symptoms all at the same time.

The GI—and its companion value, the glycemic load (GL)—are relevant *not just to you* but also your family. People with a family history of obesity, diabetes, and heart disease gain the most from putting the GI into practice. It's ideal for those who want to do the best they can to prevent these problems in the first place.

In this chapter we cover the scientific rationale of healthy low-GI eating. We also look at metabolism and the fuel hierarchy; why we need carbohydrates; how much you need; and how understanding the GI can help you choose the right amount of carbohydrates and the right type for managing PCOS.

Watch out for this symbol on foods! It's your guarantee that the GI value on the label is correct (it's been tested properly by an accredited laboratory) as well as your assurance that the food makes a nutritious contribution to the diet. Visit the Web site for more details: www.gisymbol.com.au.

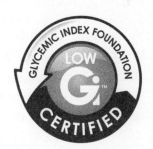

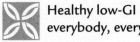 Healthy low-GI eating is for everybody, every day, every meal.

PCOS and the insulin connection

If you have PCOS, your body has a hard time bringing blood glucose levels down after you've eaten. PCOS means the body is insensitive, or you could say partially deaf, to insulin. The organs and tissues that ought to respond to even a small rise in insulin remain unresponsive. So, the body tries harder, by secreting even more insulin, to achieve the same effect, pretty much the way we all tend to raise our voice for someone who is hard of hearing. Thus high insulin levels are part and parcel of insulin resistance.

We now know that any means of improving insulin sensitivity, including drugs and weight loss, will improve symptoms of PCOS.

Many doctors have found that low-GI diets are particularly useful for women with PCOS. In addition, research is showing that low-GI diets improve weight loss, blood glucose levels, and appetite control.

Our own research in women with PCOS found that even when everything else in their diet was kept the same (e.g., the amount of carbohydrate, fat, protein, fiber, and energy), a diet based on low-GI breads and cereals improved insulin sensitivity and menstrual regularity to a greater extent than a conventional healthy diet. We also found a trend toward greater fat loss on the low GI diet, particularly in women with higher insulin levels to start with.

Low-GI diets are also consistent with all the other dietary changes needed for preventing diabetes, heart disease, and cancer, so you have nothing to lose and much to gain by following a safe, balanced, and healthy low-GI eating plan.

What you need to know about your metabolism and the fuel hierarchy

Our bodies run on fuel, just like a car runs on gas. The fuels our bodies burn are derived from a mixture of the protein, fat, carbohydrate, and alcohol that we consume. Every day we need to fill our fuel tanks with the right amount and the right kind of fuel for health, energy, and to feel our best. The actual proportions in our fuel mix will vary from hour to hour and are determined to a large extent by the last meal we ate.

There's also a fuel "hierarchy": an order of priority that our bodies follow for burning the fuels in food. Alcohol is at the top of the list because our bodies have no place to store unused alcohol (which is why it is a good idea to cut right back on alcohol if you need to lose weight). Protein comes second, followed by carbohydrate, while fat comes off last. In practice, the fuel mix is largely a combination of carbohydrate and fat in varying proportions. After meals the mix is predominantly carbohydrate and between meals it is mainly fat.

First of all let's focus on fat. The body's ability to burn all the fat we eat is one of the keys to weight control. If fat burning is inhibited, fat stores gradually accumulate. This is why the relative proportions of fat to carbohydrate in our fuel mix are critical. The proportions can vary throughout the day and are dictated by the level of insulin in the blood. For example, if our insulin levels are low, as they are when we first wake up in the morning, then the fuel mix is mainly fat. But, if our insulin levels are high, as they are after we have eaten a high-carbohydrate meal then the fuel mix we burn is mainly carbohydrate.

However, if insulin is always high, as it is if you have PCOS, then your body is constantly forced to burn carbohydrate and has trouble burning the fat that is eaten and using it as a source of fuel. When this happens, fat stores mount up. Scientists now believe that subtle abnormalities in the ability to burn fat are behind most states of being overweight or obese.

Carbohydrate is nature's primary fuel

Did you know that carbohydrate is the most widely consumed substance in the world after water? In fact, carbohydrates hold a very special place in human nutrition. Glucose, the simplest carbohydrate, is the *essential* fuel for the human brain, red blood cells, and a growing fetus, and the main source of energy for our muscles during strenuous exercise. So it makes no sense to leave it out altogether. Very low-carb diets are unnecessarily restrictive and likely to reduce your short-term mental and physical performance. They may also cause heart disease and cancer over the long term, and diets high in red meat have been linked with an increased risk of type 2 diabetes and gestational diabetes (diabetes in pregnancy). Furthermore, a large study from Harvard Medical School comparing four different diets found that a low–carb, high-protein diet was no more effective than a higher carb diet for weight loss, as long as the participants reduced their calorie intake. And the low–fat, high-carb diet resulted in the best reduction in "bad" LDL cholesterol levels. Another recent study found no benefits of a low-carb diet for weight loss or blood glucose control in people with type 2 diabetes.

Top 20 sources of carbohydrates

While sources of carbohydrate differ from country to country, most women in developed nations get their carbs from the same types of foods. In 2002, the Harvard Nurses' Health Study, which looked at the diet of more than 120,000 nurses, found that the top twenty sources of carbohydrate in their diet were:

The Pancreas Produces Insulin

The pancreas is a vital organ near the stomach. Its job is to produce the hormone insulin. Carbohydrate stimulates the secretion of insulin more than any other component of food including protein and fat. The slow absorption of the carbohydrate in low-GI foods means that the pancreas doesn't have to work so hard and produces less insulin. If the pancreas is over stimulated over a long period of time, it may become "exhausted," resulting in gestational diabetes and/or type 2 diabetes—both are common in women with a history of PCOS. Even without diabetes, high insulin levels are undesirable because they increase the risk of weight gain and heart disease.

1. Potato
2. White bread
3. Breakfast cereal
4. Dark bread (whole-grain or rye)
5. Orange juice
6. Banana
7. White rice
8. Pizza
9. Pasta
10. Muffin/cake
11. Fruit drink
12. Soft drink
13. Apple
14. Skim milk
15. Pancake
16. Table sugar
17. Jam
18. Fruit juice
19. French fries
20. Candy/confectionery

What is carbohydrate?

Carbohydrate is simply a part of food. It is the starchy part of foods like rice, bread, potatoes, and pasta. It's also the ingredient that makes foods taste sweet: the sugars in fruit and honey are carbohydrates, as are the refined sugars in soft drinks and sweets.

Carbohydrate comes mainly from plant foods, such as cereal grains, fruits, vegetables, and legumes (peas and beans). Milk products contain carbohydrate in the form of milk sugar or lactose. Lactose is the first carbohydrate we encounter as infants, and our human milk contains more lactose than any other mammal milk. It accounts for almost half the energy available to the infant.

Some foods contain a large amount of carbohydrate (cereals, potatoes, legumes, and corn are good examples), while other foods, such as string beans, broccoli, and salad greens, have very small amounts of carbohydrate. You can eat the latter freely, but they can't provide anywhere near enough carbohydrate for a moderate carbohydrate diet. And as nutritious as they can be, plain green salads aren't meals by themselves and should be complemented by a carbohydrate-dense food such as bread or legumes.

The following foods are high in carbohydrate and provide very little fat. Include them regularly in your eating plan, but spare the butter, margarine, and oil when you prepare them.

Cereal grains
These include rice, wheat, oats, barley, quinoa, rye, and anything made from them (bread, pasta, breakfast cereal, and flour). Low-GI, whole-grain types are the best choices.

Fruits
A few tasty examples are apples, oranges, bananas, grapes, and peaches.

Starchy vegetables
Foods such as corn, baby new potatoes, and sweet potato help to create filling, satisfying, low-GI meals.

Legumes
Baked beans, lentils, kidney beans, and chickpeas are excellent low-GI choices.

Milk
Not only is milk a source of carbohydrate, recent studies suggest that the calcium in dairy foods helps weight control as well as insulin resistance. Reduced-fat milks are the best choice. For those who don't eat dairy foods, calcium-fortified soy milk is a good alternative and also has a low GI (rice milk, another dairy alternative, has a high GI).

As we explained, carbohydrate is a part of food. The following list will give you an idea how much carbohydrate there is in some popular foods.

Percentage of carbohydrate

(grams per 100 grams of food) in food as eaten

apple 12%	orange 8%
baked beans 11%	pasta 70%
banana 21%	peas 8%
barley 61%	pear 12%
bread 47%	plum 6%
carrot 6%	potato 15%
cornflakes 85%	raisins 75%
cucumber 2%	rice 79%
flour 73%	split peas 45%
grapes 15%	sugar 100%
ice cream 22%	sweet potato 17%
milk 5%	sweet corn 16%
onion 5%	water cracker 71%
oats 61%	wheat cracker 62%

Carbohydrate is brain food

Unlike our muscle cells, which can burn either fat or carbohydrate, our brain does not have the "metabolic machinery" to burn fat. Unless we are literally starving (and we aren't just talking about skipping a meal or feeling very hungry here), carbohydrate is the only source of fuel that our brains can use. The brain is our most energy-demanding organ—responsible for over half our energy requirements in the resting state.

If you fast for twenty-four hours or decide not to eat carbohydrate at all, your brain will rely initially on small stores of carbohydrate in your liver. But within a few hours these will be depleted and your liver will begin synthesizing glucose from non-carbohydrate sources (including your muscle tissue). It has only a limited ability to do this, however, and any shortfall in glucose availability will have consequences for your brain function and intellectual performance.

We know from research that people perform demanding mental tasks better after eating a glucose load or carbohydrate-rich food. The mental tasks in the studies included various standard measures of "intelligence," including word recall, maze learning, arithmetic, short-term memory, rapid information processing, and reasoning. The young people, university students, people with diabetes, healthy elderly people, and people with Alzheimer's disease who took part in the studies all showed improved mental ability following a carbohydrate meal.

At all times our bodies need to maintain a minimum threshold level of glucose in the blood to serve the brain and central nervous system. If for some reason glucose levels fall below this threshold (a state called "hypoglycemia"), the consequences are severe, including trembling; dizziness; nausea; incoherent rambling speech; and lack of coordination. If not rectified, continuing hypoglycemia can lead to coma and even death. While such serious symptoms won't affect the average person, they are an ever present risk for people taking insulin or drugs to control high blood glucose levels.

What's wrong with a low-carbohydrate diet?

The low-carbohydrate diet craze has continued to get lots of attention. We are now seeing scientific studies to determine whether they work or not and what effects they may have on your long-term health. Some studies have shown that overweight people lose weight faster on a low-carbohydrate diet than on a high-carbohydrate one. Furthermore, there were no obvious adverse effects over the short term. But others have shown no benefit over a higher-carb diet.

When I passed a really important exam at my ballet school, my family and I decided we'd all go out to a club in town to celebrate. I hadn't eaten much that day as I had been really busy, just a slice of toast with peanut butter at lunchtime. My sister and I sneaked a small drink before we left and then at the club I probably overdid it—I had six gin cocktails over two hours. I don't remember snacking while I was drinking. The next thing I do remember is waking up in the emergency room of the local hospital, with an intravenous line delivering 5 percent glucose. I had passed out in the club and was "unresponsive." The ambulance crew found my blood glucose drawn from a finger prick was really low (less than 2 mmol /L). The next day I was discharged, apparently no worse for wear, and told to go and see my doctor, who referred me to an endocrinologist because of the low blood glucose. The doctor asked me lots of questions and I recalled feeling a bit light-headed and sweaty on a few occasions in recent months. All the tests, however, showed nothing unusual at all. That's when the endocrinologist suggested to Mom and me that, as a long shot, he would check me out for PCOS (which I had never heard of) as a possible underlying cause of insulin resistance. This time the tests came back positive. It was such a relief to find out what the matter was. I was prescribed metformin and put on a diet plan of healthy low-GI eating, including lots of vegetables, pasta, whole-grain bread, and legumes. And, of course, was advised not to drink too much alcohol and, if I am out having a drink with friends, to make sure I have something to eat. I have to say I have become a real enthusiast for my new diet and I haven't missed a single dose of metformin. After two and a half years, despite a very active social life, I haven't experienced another episode of symptomatic low blood glucose, which apparently is very rare.

Melissa, 18

There are also some real concerns with very low-carbohydrate diets. They may help lower insulin levels temporarily, but their high saturated fat content may be causing lots of ill effects in the longer term. Indeed, high levels of saturated fats are associated with insulin resistance and heart disease. Recent studies have shown that low–carb, high-protein diets may worsen blood vessel function, which could increase heart disease risk. There is also now a significant amount of evidence to show that diets high in red meat (as most high-protein, low-carb diets tend to be) are linked with an increased risk of type 2 diabetes and gestational diabetes.

Keeping that in mind, high-carbohydrate diets may not be the optimal way to lose weight either, particularly if the carbs are not low GI. If they raise your blood glucose and insulin levels, then it's no surprise that burning body fat will be twice as hard. Low-carbohydrate diets may be effective in the short term because they lower glucose and insulin levels. So the answer is probably somewhere in the middle—a moderate carbohydrate intake, coming mostly from low GI carbs, and moderate increase in protein, focusing on more plant protein rather than animal protein. In fact a recent study found that a low-carbohydrate diet based on animal sources was associated with an increased mortality, whereas a vegetable-based low-carbohydrate diet was associated with a lower risk of mortality from all causes and cardiovascular disease.

For the first half of the last century, people with diabetes were told to follow low-carbohydrate diets (to keep their blood glucose levels down) and to get their calories from high protein fatty foods. Trouble was, they were dying early of heart attack, rather than diabetes.

When cautious studies were carried out with high-carbohydrate diets, doctors were stunned to find that blood glucose control improved and blood fats came down. Nowadays, after much research, people with diabetes are advised to follow a moderately high-carbohydrate diet. Most people also find low-carbohydrate diets are hard to live with because they cut out so many of the foods that we love: bread, fruit, potatoes, pasta, to name just a few. It's not so surprising that people lose weight on such a limited diet. And it's even less surprising that they find it hard to stick to. Women with PCOS need to take a long-term view of their health—it's not just a few weeks of weight loss but a whole new way of eating to reduce your chances of developing diabetes or heart disease.

For weight control—not just in the short term but keeping it off for good—you need to follow an eating plan that you love.

The bottom line is that the *type* of carbohydrate and the type of fat are more critical than the precise *amount*. Choosing low-GI carbs will not only assist with weight control, it will reduce blood glucose and insulin levels throughout the day, increase your sense of feeling full and satisfied, and provide bulk and a rich supply of micronutrients including zinc, calcium, and magnesium. All these factors work together to increase insulin sensitivity and improve the signs and symptoms of PCOS.

 Unlike low-carbohydrate diets, low-GI diets are safe, balanced, and provide all the micronutrients for optimum health.

How much carbohydrate do we need?

As we have shown, there are good reasons to avoid a low-carbohydrate diet (less than 30 percent of energy as carbs), but what then is the optimal level of carbohydrate in the diet? Should it be as high as 65 percent of total daily calories, as some nutritionists and doctors recommend, or a more moderate 45 percent of energy?

The American Institute of Medicine published the most recent nutritional guidelines in 2002 (new guidelines are due in late 2010). Their recommendations indicate that both moderate and high levels (45–65 percent of energy) or anything in between can work to meet the body's daily energy and nutritional needs while minimizing the risk for chronic disease. And if we look carefully at diets around the world, it's clear that both high and moderate intakes of carbohydrate are commensurate with good health. The only group of people who naturally follow a low-carbohydrate diet are traditional-living Eskimos (Inuits), who eat large amounts of protein and unsaturated fat from seafood.

Our approach is that your carbohydrate intake can be either high or moderate, as long as you give due consideration to the type of foods you eat. It may be helpful to discuss your own particular needs and food preferences with a registered dietitian (RD).

Is a high-carbohydrate diet for you?

Most of the world's population currently eats a high carbohydrate diet based on staples such as rice, corn, millet, and wheat-based foods like bread or noodles. In some African and Asian countries, for example, carbohydrate may form as much as 70–80 percent of a person's energy intake—but this is probably too high for optimum health. In contrast, people in industrialized nations such as the United States, Australia, New Zealand, and the UK eat less than half of their calories as carbohydrates; typically only 40–45 percent carbohydrate. A high-carbohydrate diet has more than 50 percent of energy as carbohydrate.

Is consuming at least half of your total daily calories as carbohydrate realistic for you? That depends. If you have always been health conscious and avoided high-fat foods, or if you enjoy an Asian-style diet most of the time, then chances are you're already eating a high-carbohydrate diet. If this is the case, the key for you is to switch your carbs to lower GI choices.

Of course, the number of calories, and hence the amount of carbohydrate, varies with your weight and activity levels. If you are an active person with average energy requirements who is not trying to lose weight (i.e., with an average intake of 2,000 calories per day), you will eat 275 grams of carbohydrate. If you are trying to lose weight and are consuming a low-calorie diet (i.e., a small eater on 1,200 calories per day), it means eating about 165 grams of carbohydrate a day.

Is a moderate-carbohydrate diet for you?

A Mediterranean-style diet that includes olive oil and nuts is higher in fat and provides only about 45 percent of energy as carbohydrate. In the past, dietitians and nutritionists here and countries like Australia, New Zealand, and the UK would have frowned upon this, but that's no longer the case. We now know that as long as you carefully consider the types of fats and the types of carbohydrate, then this amount of carbohydrate is perfectly compatible with good health. At this level, you need to consume at least 125 grams of carbohydrate a day if you are a small eater and 225 grams if you are an average eater.

 Today's health recommendations are as much about the type of fat and the nature of the carbohydrate as about the total amounts of each.

In the end, the choice of how much carbohydrate you eat—moderate or high—is yours. Our approach has built-in flexibility when it comes to the amount of carbohydrate you need to eat. It's not rocket science to suggest that the way of eating that you'll enjoy and tend to follow over the long term is the one that is closest to your usual diet and to your cultural and ethnic origins. What we emphasize is that the *type* or *source* of the carbohydrate and fat are just as important as the amount. We believe that, unlike baseball caps, one size does not fit all.

The GI: the real deal on carbohydrates

It's time to look at the type or nature of the carbohydrate in your diet. The most important thing to keep in mind is that all carbohydrates were not created equal—you must choose the right kind of carbohydrate for your lifestyle.

Traditionally, the nature of carbohydrates was described by their chemical structure: simple or complex. Sugars were simple and starches were complex, simply because sugars were small molecules and starches were big. By virtue of their large size, it was automatically assumed that complex carbohydrates, such as starches, would be slowly digested and absorbed by our bodies and would cause only a small and gradual rise in blood glucose levels. Simple sugars, on the other hand, were assumed to be the villains, being digested and absorbed quickly, producing a rapid rise in blood glucose.

A few very elementary experiments long ago on raw starches and pure sugars seemed to support these assumptions, and for fifty years they were taught to every medical and biochemistry student as "fact."

We now know that the whole chemical concept of "simple" versus "complex" carbohydrate does not tell us anything about how the carbohydrates in our food change blood glucose levels in our bodies.

Thirty years of scientific research with real people and real food have shown that those assumptions about the speed of digestion were all wrong.

The rise in blood glucose after meals could not be predicted simply on the basis of a simple versus complex chemical structure. Another system of describing the nature of carbohydrates and classifying them according to their effects on blood glucose was needed: the glycemic index served that purpose.

It may seem surprising today, but scientists did not study the actual blood glucose responses to common foods in real people until the early 1980s. Since 1981, nearly two thousand different foods have been tested as single foods and in mixed meals with both healthy people and people with diabetes. Professors David Jenkins and Tom Wolever at the University of Toronto were the first to introduce the term "glycemic index" to compare the ability of different carbohydrates to raise blood glucose levels.

The GI is simply a numerical way of describing how the carbohydrates in individual foods affect blood glucose levels. Foods with a high GI value contain carbohydrates that cause a dramatic rise in blood glucose levels, while foods with a low GI value contain carbohydrates with much less impact. This research has turned some widely held beliefs upside down.

How to Find a Dietitian

For specific information about your own calorie and exact carbohydrate needs, you should consult a registered dietitian (RD). Look in the *Yellow Pages* under Dietitians or call the American Dietetic Association's Consumer Nutrition Hotline (800–366–1655) or go to the ADA's home page: http://www.eatright.org. Make sure that the person you choose has the letters RD after his or her name.

 The GI is a measure of how fast carbohydrates hit the bloodstream. It compares carbohydrates weight for weight, gram for gram.

The first surprise was that the starch in foods like bread, potatoes, and many types of rice is digested and absorbed very quickly, not slowly, as had always been assumed.

Second, scientists found that the sugar in foods (like fruit, confectionery, and ice cream) did not produce more rapid or prolonged rises in blood glucose, as had always been thought. The truth was that most of the sugars in foods, regardless of the source, actually produced quite moderate blood glucose responses, lower than most starches.

So we all need to forget the old distinctions that have been made between starchy foods and sugary foods, or simple versus complex carbohydrates. They have no useful application when it comes to blood glucose levels. Even an experienced scientist with a detailed knowledge of a food's chemical composition finds it difficult to predict a food's GI value.

 Forget about the words simple and complex carbohydrate. Think in terms of low and high GI values.

The key to understanding the GI is the rate of digestion

Foods containing carbohydrates that break down quickly during digestion have the highest GI values. The blood glucose response is fast and high. In other words, the glucose (or sugar) in the bloodstream increases rapidly. Conversely, foods that contain carbohydrates that break down slowly, releasing glucose gradually into the bloodstream, have a low GI value.

An analogy we like to use is the popular fable of the tortoise and the hare. The hare, just like high-GI foods, speeds away but loses the race to the tortoise with his slow and steady pace. Similarly, slow and steady low-GI foods produce a smooth blood glucose curve without wild fluctuations. The graph below shows the different effects of slow and fast carbohydrates on our blood glucose levels.

For most people, foods with low GI values have advantages over those with high GI values; however, in elite sport, there are times when a high-GI food will be the best choice.

The substance that produces one of the greatest effects on blood glucose levels is pure glucose itself. GI testing has shown that most

Measuring the GI of a Food

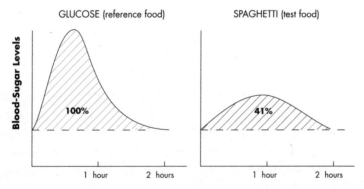

The test food and the reference food must contain the same amount of carbohydrate. The usual dose is 50 grams, but sometimes 25 grams is used when the portion size would be otherwise too large. Even smaller doses such as 15 grams have been used. The GI result is much the same whatever the dose because the GI is simply a relative measure of carbohydrate quality.

foods have less effect on blood glucose levels than glucose (also called dextrose). The GI value of pure glucose is set at 100 and every other food is ranked on a scale from 0 to 100 according to the actual effect on blood glucose levels. (Note: There are a few foods that have GI values of more than 100, e.g., jasmine rice. While this seems extraordinary, there's a simple explanation. Glucose is a highly concentrated solution that tends to be held up briefly in the stomach. On the other hand, jasmine rice contains starch that leaves the stomach without delay and is then digested at lightning speed.)

 The glycemic index is a clinically proven tool in its applications to diabetes and weight control.

What determines a food's GI?

Everyone wants to know what gives one food a high GI value and another one a low GI value. There is a wealth of information, which can easily confuse. We have summarized in simple terms the results of the most recent scientific research in the table on pages 41–42, which looks at the various factors that influence the GI value of a food.

The key message is that the physical state of the starch in a food is by far the most important factor influencing its GI value. That's why the advances in food processing over the past two hundred years have had such a profound effect on the overall GI values of the carbohydrates we eat.

The GI was never meant to be used in isolation!

At first glance when you look at a list of foods with a low GI value it might appear that some high-fat foods such as chocolate seem a good choice simply because they have a low GI value. This is absolutely not the case. A food's GI value was never meant to be the only criterion by which it is judged. Large amounts of fat (and protein) in food tend to slow the rate of stomach emptying and therefore the rate at which foods are digested in the small intestine.

High, medium, or low GI . . .

A high GI value is 70 or more
A medium GI level is 56–69 inclusive
A low GI value is 55 or less

High-fat foods will therefore tend to have lower GI values than their low-fat equivalents. For example, potato chips have a lower GI value (54) than potatoes baked without fat (85).

Many biscuits have a lower GI value (40–60) than bread (70). In these instances, a lower GI value doesn't mean an automatically better choice from a nutritional standpoint. Saturated fat in these foods will have adverse effects on coronary health, far greater than the benefit of lower blood glucose levels. These foods should be treated as "indulgences."

This is not to say that all fats in foods should be avoided. One of the reasons why nuts have such a low GI value is their relatively high fat content compared to cereal grains. But just as there are differences in the nature of carbohydrates in foods, there are differences in the quality of fats. We need to be choosy about fats too. Healthy fats, such as the omega-3 polyunsaturated fats, are not only good for us, they help to lower the blood glucose response to meals.

The right kind of carbohydrate

Both high and moderate carbohydrate intake can be healthy—the choice is simply up to you. Both types of diets, however, need to emphasize low-GI carbohydrates and healthy fats.

To ensure that you are eating enough carbohydrate and the right kind, you should eat:

- fruits for snacks or dessert: aim for 2–3 pieces per day
- vegetables with lunch and dinner and even as snacks: aim for at least five servings per day
- at least one low-GI food at each meal: aim for four servings of whole-grain cereals per day
- lots of fiber (foods with low energy density or fewer calories per gram)

Digesting Carbohydrates

To make use of the sugars and starches in foods, our bodies first have to break them down into a form that we can absorb and that our bodies can use. This is what we call digestion.

Digestion starts in the mouth where the starch-digesting enzyme in our saliva, which is called amylase, is incorporated into our food as we chew. Amylase chops up long-chain starch molecules into short-chain molecules such as maltose and maltodextrins. Its activity is halted by the acids secreted into the stomach and most digestion continues only when the carbohydrate leaves the stomach and reaches the small intestine.

The rate at which food enters the small intestine from the stomach is called the rate of stomach (or gastric) emptying. Some food components—such as viscous or "sticky" fiber, acidic compounds such as vinegar, and very concentrated solutions—help to slow down stomach emptying and therefore the overall speed of carbohydrate digestion.

In the small intestine, starch digestion continues. Huge amounts of amylase are secreted in pancreatic juice into the small intestine, so much so that the biochemists call it amylase "overkill." The speed of digestion now depends on the nature of the starch itself—how resistant it is in a physical and chemical sense to being attacked by enzymes. Many starches in food are rapidly digested, while others are more resistant and the process is slower.

Other food factors may influence the speed of digestion. If the mixture of food and enzymes is highly viscous or sticky, owing to the presence of viscous fiber, mixing slows down and the enzymes and starch take longer to make contact. The products of starch digestion will also take longer to move toward the wall of the intestine, where the last steps in digestion take place.

At the intestinal wall, the short-chain starch products, together with the sugars in foods, are broken down by specific enzymes. The monosaccharides that finally result from starch and sugar digestion include glucose, fructose, and galactose. They are absorbed from the small intestine into the bloodstream, where they are available as a source of energy to the cells.

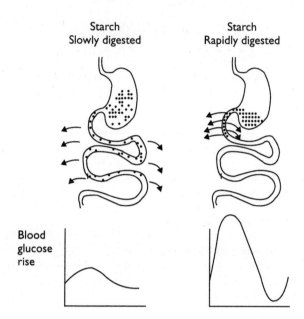

You will find that when you are choosy about your carbohydrates, your insulin levels will be lower and you will automatically burn more fat. You may not feel this change as it is happening, but you will see the results over time (you'll lose weight!). Eating high-fiber foods will also help fill you up and prevent you from overeating.

The right kind of fat

For most people, "low fat" is still synonymous with "healthy" and "weight loss." Forget it! Once upon a time, when fruits, vegetables, and whole grains were the staples of a low-fat diet, it might have been true.

But it is no longer so—indeed, the typical low-fat diet may be distinctly unhealthy and one of the reasons behind our expanding waistlines. In the 1990s, the experts told us to eat low-fat diets because they were concerned about two things. First, saturated fat increases the risk of heart disease; second, fatty foods are too easily overeaten because they are energy-dense. Those concerns are still valid today. But the solution to the problem—recommending a low-fat diet—has not been a successful strategy. While we've cut down on total fat, we haven't cut down on saturated fat, and the food industry (with the best intentions) gave us a myriad of low-fat foods that were

Factors that influence the GI value of a food

FACTOR	MECHANISM	EXAMPLES OF FOOD WHERE THE EFFECT IS SEEN
Starch gelatinization	The less gelatinized (swollen) the starch, the slower the rate of digestion.	Al dente spaghetti, oatmeal, and biscuits have less gelatinized starch.
Physical entrapment	The fibrous coat around beans and seeds and plant cell walls acts as a physical barrier, slowing down access of enzymes to the starch inside.	Pumpernickel and grainy bread, legumes, and barley.
High amylose to amylopectin ratio*	The more amylose a food contains, the less water the starch will absorb and the slower its rate of digestion.	Basmati rice and legumes contain more amylose than other cereals.
Particle size	The smaller the particle size, the easier it is for water and enzymes to penetrate.	Finely milled flours have high GI values. Stone ground flours have larger particles and lower GIs.
Viscosity of fiber	Viscous, soluble fibers increase the viscosity of the intestinal contents and this slows down the interaction between the starch and the enzymes.	Finely milled wheat and rye flours have fast rates of digestion and absorption because the fiber is not fibrous. Rolled oats, beans, lentils, apples, Metamucil.
Sugar	The digestion of sugar produces only half as many glucose molecules as the same amount of starch (the other half is fructose). The presence of sugar also restricts gelatinization of the starch by binding water and reducing the amount of "available" water.	Social Tea Biscuits, oatmeal biscuits, and some breakfast cereals (Kellogg's Frosted Flakes) that are high in sugar have relatively low GI values.

(continues)

(continued)

Factors that influence the GI value of a food

FACTOR	MECHANISM	EXAMPLES OF FOOD WHERE THE EFFECT IS SEEN
Acidity	Acids in food slow down stomach emptying, thereby slowing the rate at which starch can be digested.	Vinegar, lemon juice, lime juice, some salad dressings, pickled vegetables, and sourdough bread.
Fat	Fat slows down the rate of stomach emptying, thereby slowing the digestion of the starch.	Potato chips have a lower GI value than boiled white potatoes.

* Amylose and amylopectin are two different types of starch. Both are found in foods, but the ratio varies.

The Effect of Starch Gelatinization on the Glycemic Index

The starch in raw food is stored in hard, compact granules that make it difficult to digest. Most starchy foods need to be cooked for this reason. During cooking, water and heat expand the starch granules to different degrees; some granules actually burst and the individual starch molecules release. This process is called gelatinization.

The swollen granules and free starch molecules are very easy to digest. The quick action of the enzymes results in a rapid, high blood glucose rise after consumption. A food containing starch that is fully gelatinized will therefore have a very high GI value.

just as energy-dense as their full-fat counterparts. So during the 1990s, the era of "99 percent fat free," the prevalence of obesity soared, and, with it, heart disease and diabetes.

As a result of these unexpected events, the American Heart Association went back to the drawing board in 2000 and again in 2006 to

Glycemic Load

Glycemic load provides a measure of the degree of glycemia and insulin demand produced by a normal serving of the food. Glycemic load is calculated simply by multiplying the GI of a food by the amount of carbohydrate per serving and dividing by 100.

Glycemic load = (GI × carbohydrate per serving) ÷ 100.

The glycemic load is greatest for those foods that provide the most carbohydrate, particularly those we tend to eat in large quantities. Some nutritionists have argued that the glycemic load is an improvement on the GI because it provides an estimate of both quantity and quality of carbohydrate (the GI gives us just quality). In large-scale studies from Harvard University, however, the risk of disease was predicted by both the GI of the overall diet as well as the glycemic load. The use of the glycemic load strengthened the relationship, suggesting that the more frequent the consumption of high-carbohydrate, high-GI foods, the more adverse the health outcome.

Don't make the mistake of using GL alone. If you do, you might find yourself eating a diet with very little carbohydrate but a lot of fat, especially saturated fat, and excessive amounts of protein. Use the glycemic index to compare foods of similar nature (e.g., bread with bread) and use the glycemic load when you note a high GI but low carbohydrate content per serving (e.g., pumpkin).

You'll find both the GI and GL of many foods later in this book (see pages 181–222).

remodel their dietary advice. The dietary guidelines now stress the importance of preventing obesity and are easier to use. Their strategy promotes an overall healthy eating plan for Americans that includes achieving a healthy body weight, rather than focusing on a percentage of calories to be consumed from dietary fat and other nutrients. Eating a varied diet full of fruits, vegetables, whole grains, fish, poultry, lean meats, fat-free and low-fat dairy products, and including "good fats" in our diets is their focus—while still limiting foods with a high content of saturated fat, cholesterol, and trans-fatty acids.

Furthermore, most of us need to eat *more* of certain kinds of fat for optimal health (yes, you read it right). These include the omega-3 fats found in fish, canola-based products, and omega-3 enriched eggs. Eating these and more monounsaturated fats like those in olive oil and canola oil has been shown to significantly reduce the risk of a heart attack. Indeed, one of the most important diet studies ever carried out, the Lyon Heart study, showed that this type of diet (with more fish, fruit, veggies, and good fats) was twice as effective in reducing the risk of another heart attack as the standard low-fat diet previously recommended by the American Heart Association.

There's another excellent reason why you should aim to increase these fats at the expense of the saturated ones. While all fats have the same number of calories per gram, they may not all have the same effect on your weight. For reasons that are not yet clear, a weight-loss diet that emphasizes fish or monounsaturated fats like olive oil is much more likely to reduce abdominal body fat. This is a critical point for women with PCOS whose excess fat around the waist is directly linked to their insulin resistance. If they can reduce that stubborn fat, insulin levels will come down and hence reduce signs and symptoms of PCOS.

Where do you find the good fats?

- fish such as salmon, tuna, herrings, sardines—canned or fresh—but any fish is better than none at all (see page 96 for more information on fish)
- shellfish, prawns, scallops
- walnuts, almonds, cashews—best unsalted, forget the chips and salty snacks
- avocado—spread it on bread as an alternative to margarine or butter
- olives—spread as a tapenade or add whole to almost anything—pasta sauces or salads
- muesli—mix sunflowers seeds, pumpkin seeds, ground almond, or hazelnuts
- flaxseed is a great source of omega-3 fats: try flaxseed bread or using flaxseed oil in salad dressings

There are two important things to remember in improving your diet:

1. Identify the sources of carbohydrate in your diet and reduce high-GI foods. Don't go to extremes; there is room for your favorite high-GI foods.

2. Identify the sources of fat and look at ways you can reduce saturated fat. Choose monounsaturated and polyunsaturated fats, such as olive oil and sunflower oil, instead of saturated fats like butter and shortening. Again, don't go overboard—the body needs some fat, and there's room for your favorite fatty foods on occasion.

What about protein?

Incorporating more protein in our diet makes good sense for weight control. Protein is the best in terms of satiety—that pleasant feeling of fullness after eating. In comparison with carbohydrate and fat, protein makes us feel more satisfied immediately after eating and reduces hunger between meals. That's critically important because hunger makes or breaks a diet and compromises long-term weight control. Protein also increases our metabolic rate during the hour or two after eating. We burn more energy by the minute compared with the increase that occurs after eating carbs or fats. Even though this is a relatively small difference it may be important in long-term weight control. Lastly, protein foods are excellent sources of micronutrients, such as iron, zinc, vitamin B_{12}, and omega-3 fats. So, even though you're cutting energy intake, you're not cutting good nutrition.

Most of us obtain about 15 percent of the energy in our diet from protein. If you wish (it's up to you) you can increase this to as much as 30 percent without cause for concern. Recent studies show that this higher level increases the rate of weight and body fat loss, at least in the short term. In a similar way to carbohydrate and fat, the *source* of extra protein is critical. Lean meats (beef, pork, lamb), chicken, fish, and shellfish are ideal. Go for the leanest cuts in the supermarket—grill, stir-fry, or barbeque, and cut off all the visible fat.

Good plant-based protein sources include tofu, tempeh, quorn, and TVP as well as legumes (which are also a good source of low-GI carbs), nuts, and seeds (which also supply healthy fats). These are all versatile ingredients that can be enjoyed in a variety of dishes for vegetarians and nonvegetarians alike.

Dairy products are more than good sources of protein—the combination of protein and calcium that's unique to dairy appears to aid weight control. Studies have shown that the more calcium or dairy (it's hard to separate the two) people eat, the lower their weight and fat mass. Calcium is known to be intimately involved in the burning of fat—and that's something we want to encourage! However, we have to be a little selective about which dairy foods we eat. Choose low-fat dairy products including milk, yogurt, and cheese.

Nuts are also excellent sources of protein, dietary fiber, and micronutrients, and eating nuts regularly has been linked with a reduced risk of type 2 diabetes and heart disease.

Finally, eggs are great sources of protein and essential vitamins and minerals. If you select the "omega-3" eggs on the market, you will also boost the good fats in your diet.

 Not all carbohydrates were created equal—you must choose the right kind of carbohydrate for your lifestyle.

Chapter 2 in a nutshell

Let's sum up the main points we've covered in this chapter.

- There are sound reasons to eat a moderately high carbohydrate diet if you have PCOS.
- Low-carb diets are unnecessarily restrictive and may be harmful in the long term.
- The nature of the carbohydrate is more important than the absolute amount.
- Low-GI carbs lower insulin levels and improve insulin sensitivity, the key to beating PCOS.
- Low-GI carbs are more satiating and help reduce hunger between meals, the key to long-term weight control.

- The kind of fat is more important than the amount: reduce saturated fat, increase the good fats.
- Higher protein intakes may be helpful to weight control.

Chapter 8 offers the glycemic index values and glycemic load of over 1,300 popular foods.

In the next chapter, we show you exactly what you need to do and eat to put it all into practice.

3

Four Steps to Taking Charge

WHEN WE TALK TO WOMEN with PCOS the one thing they tell us time and again is that they feel "out of control"—gaining weight, being unable to fall pregnant, and growing an excessive amount of body hair in areas where it just shouldn't be. We have found that by showing these women how to make some basic lifestyle changes, such as eating the right kinds of food and exercising more, they can start to feel in control of their lives again. In fact, by following our diet and exercise suggestions many women have found that they can take charge of their health in a way they never have before, and can effectively manage their PCOS symptoms.

We started this book by describing, as simply as we could, what PCOS is, the insulin connection, and why what you eat plays such an important part in helping you manage PCOS symptoms. It's time now to show you how you can make the change to low-GI healthy eating and build more exercise into your life. This chapter shares the four steps to taking charge and is packed with plenty of practical ideas you can implement right now.

The real benefits we have seen with many women and girls who have adopted a healthy low-GI way of eating and stepped up the exercise and activity schedule include:

- improving PCOS symptoms—regulating menstrual cycles, reducing acne and excess hair growth
- achieving and maintaining a healthy weight
- controlling blood glucose and insulin levels
- balancing hormone levels
- boosting fertility
- gaining control and quality of life

And if pregnancy is one of your plans for the future, making these lifestyle changes can lead to dramatic improvements in ovulation, pregnancy rates, and reducing the risk of miscarriage.

At the same time, you will also be going a long way toward reducing your risk of developing type 2 diabetes and heart disease.

By the way, when we use the word "diet" we're talking about eating the healthy low-GI way, not about those restrictive diets that we know don't work in the long term.

The four steps

Be reassured, we aren't going to ask you to work out on a treadmill for hours on end, starve yourself, or try and remember long food lists of dos and don'ts. Quite the opposite. Our program is based on little changes that you can easily incorporate into your life and that you will feel comfortable with. In addition, we can promise that you won't feel hungry and, if you stick to it, you'll have more energy. What's more, we don't expect you to do everything at once. One step at a time is fine. The four basic steps to taking charge of your PCOS symptoms the low-GI way are:

- managing your weight
- eating a healthy low-GI diet
- moving more
- taking care of yourself

Managing your weight

Managing your weight is really important if you have PCOS. Being overweight increases insulin resistance, worsens the symptoms of PCOS, and increases the risk of developing diabetes as you get older. The good news is that you don't need to lose a lot of weight (or body fat) to start improving your PCOS symptoms.

We now know from the women we have helped and from many scientific studies that losing as little as 5 percent of body weight can help control blood glucose levels, improve menstrual function, reduce testosterone levels, improve an excess hair problem, and help with acne. So how much weight does this actually mean? Well, if you are 220 pounds this means that losing around 11 pounds of body fat can make a difference, and if you are 154 pounds as little as 8 pounds can help you to start taking control. In the long term, you should aim to lose 10 percent of your current body weight—this will go a long way toward reducing or even reversing your insulin resistance.

It makes sense that achieving and maintaining a healthy weight comes from balancing your energy intake from the food you eat with your energy output from whatever physical activity you do. So, when you take in more energy from food than you burn up, you tend to put on weight or, rather, store fat. To lose weight and shed that fat, you need to eat less or move more—and it's pretty obvious that the most effective way is to do some of both.

Here's the really important part: when we talk about eating less, we don't mean starving yourself and feeling hungry all the time. We mean choosing the right foods, the ones that the body burns rather than stores as fat and that satisfy the appetite for breakfast, lunch, dinner, and snacks in between. This is where the glycemic index and eating the healthy low-GI way comes in.

To whet your appetite, just imagine breakfasts such as Quaker creamy, old-fashioned oatmeal with dried fruit and yogurt, whole wheat blueberry pancakes, or sweet corn, bacon, and mushroom omelets with whole-grain toast. Or main meals like pasta with roasted sweet potato and feta cheese, bean and corn burritos, or lamb burgers. And for dessert there is cherry strudel, apple and rhubarb crumble with muesli and walnut topping, or baked ricotta cheese-cake. Hungry? You can enjoy all these foods and more when you take control and start managing your weight by eating well and moving more. In our experience, when women change to a healthy low-GI diet they often comment on the fact that they are feeling fuller and are less tempted to snack on those "not so healthy" energy-dense foods—a big help when you are trying to lose weight.

Avoiding the dreaded yoyo dieting cycle

If you want to lose body fat and keep it off, restrictive dieting isn't the answer. Calorie counting may help you lose "weight" (on the scales), but doesn't necessarily help you lose body fat. And it's almost impossible for most people to stick to in the long term.

What happens when you go on a restrictive diet is that you starve the body of carbohydrates and use up the carbohydrate stores (glycogen) in the muscles. As every gram of glycogen is stored along with 3 grams of water, the initial fast drop in weight you see on the scales is mainly due to water loss. Once you have used up the glycogen stores in your muscles, the body breaks down some of its own muscle tissue to supply glucose to the brain. Lean muscle tissue, unlike fat, is active—it uses up energy even when you are at rest. Losing muscle tissue therefore slows down your metabolism, which means the body needs less energy to do the same work it used to. And this is how the dreaded yoyo dieting cycle begins.

The human body is also extremely good at adapting to the amount of energy we give it and this is what happens when you starve your body with a restrictive diet. First your body tries to conserve energy, slowing down your metabolism. Then, as soon as you go off that restrictive diet (which, if you are like most people, is pretty inevitable), you will probably pile the weight you have just lost right back on, plus a bit extra because your body now needs less energy to survive than it used to. So, if you go on and off diets, your body ends up with less and less muscle and more and more fat, which is why restrictive dieting can make you fat.

In the end, most restrictive diets don't work because they are just too hard to stick to for any length of time. If you are hungry and tired all the time, or if what you have to eat on your restrictive diet

Low GI and Weight Regain

Many people who successfully lose weight find themselves gradually putting the weight back on. Scientists are now focusing on this critical period, trying to determine the optimal dietary strategy for maintaining weight loss and preventing weight regain. The findings of the largest study of its kind, the Diogenes Study, led by Professor Arne Astrup at the University of Copenhagen, are just beginning to emerge. This collaborative project from eight countries in the European Union included over 800 overweight or obese individuals, all of them parents of young children. One or two parents in each family underwent an eight-week weight-loss diet using a low-calorie diet formula, which was designed to achieve a weight loss of 8 percent of their original starting weight (about twenty-four pounds). If the parents were successful in meeting this target, they were offered the opportunity to participate in the next stage of the study, which investigated the problem of weight regain. In this part of the study, volunteers were assigned to one of five different dietary regimes, designed to test the relative effectiveness of the GI as well as protein content in weight control. The diets were:

Group 1: Low protein, low glycemic index
Group 2: Low protein, high glycemic index
Group 3: High protein, low glycemic index
Group 4: High protein, high glycemic index
Group 5: Control diet, medium protein, and medium glycemic index

Over the course of twelve months, the investigators found that both low-GI diets *and* high-protein diets were equally effective in preventing weight regain (see figure 8). But they also found something that took them by complete surprise. The third diet group who combined both low GI *and* high-protein strategies continued to lose weight throughout the one-year follow-up. This was something never seen before in any study of weight maintenance after weight loss. Furthermore, this group had the lowest dropout rate of any of the groups, a testament to the fact that not only was this diet effective, but it was also acceptable to the volunteers and their families—not too difficult, complex, or hard to sustain. Interestingly, the Diogenes Study achieved only a moderately small reduction in GI (from about 58 to 50), yet it was sufficient to produce these outstanding results. It is also important to note that the high-protein diets in this study

(continues)

Low GI and Weight Regain *(continued)*

were not the very low-carb Atkins-style diets—protein provided around 25 percent of energy but these groups still ate 45 to 50 percent of their energy from carbs.

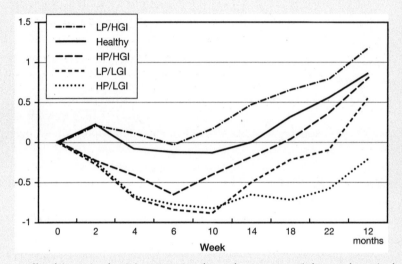

All subjects in the Diogenes Study underwent an eight-week period of fast weight loss before starting on one of five dietary strategies to prevent weight regain. (Week 0 in the figure represents the end of the eight-week period.) The two low-GI diet groups continued to lose weight in the first six months, but the best outcome after twelve months was the combination of a low-GI and high-protein diet (HP/LGI in the figure).

doesn't fit in with your family and social life, you may see the weight drop off in the first few weeks, but you are unlikely to stick with the diet long term.

So, what's the healthy way to lose weight?

Here are some tips on the healthy way to help you lose weight and keep it off long term.

Ever Heard Someone Say "I Have a Slow Metabolism" or "She's Lucky, She Has a Fast Metabolism?"

Here's what that really means. Your resting metabolic rate—the amount of energy you burn at rest—largely determines your ability to lose or gain weight. The lower your metabolic rate, the greater the tendency you have to gain weight. Your metabolic rate depends largely on the amount of muscle you have, so building muscle through exercise is an important part of weight control. Excessive dieting and overly restricting our food intake can reduce our metabolic rate. Eating the healthy low-GI way and moving more both help you to maintain a high metabolism. And that's important.

First of all, aim to lose body fat rather than weight. Put the scales away and get out the tape measure. It's more useful to go by how your clothes fit. If your body is fit and toned, who cares what it weighs?

Don't think about going on a restrictive diet. The only way to lose weight and body fat permanently is to change your eating habits and include regular physical activity in your day. This can mean changing the habits of a lifetime, so don't expect miracles of yourself. The key is to make gradual changes that will fit in with your lifestyle and last a lifetime.

It is really important to be patient and have realistic expectations. Think about how long it took to put that weight on. Twelve months? Two years? Don't expect to lose it overnight. There's no magic bullet. Losing body fat is a slow and steady business, but it's much more likely to be permanent.

Moderation is the key. There is no need to avoid any foods totally if you enjoy them—all foods can be included as part of a healthy eating plan. Obviously you need to set some limits, but cutting out all your favorite foods and feeling guilty about eating is not the way to go. Remember, your new eating plan needs to be for life. It means eating right, not necessarily less.

But none of this will work if you don't get moving. It's essential to include some regular physical activity in your day. It's not only important for weight management; it's good for your heart, your bones, for reducing diabetes risk, and for managing stress.

 Don't diet. Focus on eating well and moving more. Enjoy the foods you eat and make sure you choose the ones that will give you energy to burn. And remember, we all need to be active every day.

5 Steps to Developing Good Eating Habits

1. Listen to your appetite and avoid nonhungry eating—this is the eating you do when bored, stressed, or upset. Find alternative ways of coping with these feelings rather than heading for the fridge. You need to find other activities that provide you with the pleasure you get from food—write yourself a list!
2. Focus on what you should eat rather than what you shouldn't— if you fill up on the foods your body needs each day, there won't be much room left for the rest! Eating small amounts often and choosing foods that are satisfying will also help—this is where the GI is important as low-GI foods generally keep you fuller for longer.
3. Relax and enjoy your meals, eat slowly, and always sit down to eat—you are more likely to be satisfied if you do. Try to avoid eating on the run and get out of the habit of eating while you are doing other things such as watching TV or working.
4. Stock your cupboards with the foods you plan to eat (see pages 114-116 for your healthy low-GI shopping list) and avoid buying the foods you want to eat less of. This will be easier if you shop with a list and not when you are hungry!
5. Don't try to change everything overnight or cut out all your favorite foods—this is not sustainable! It is much easier to make one or two changes at a time and to still include a little of what you enjoy.

What Happens When You See a Dietitian?

Seeing a dietitian is not about being given a list of foods you can't eat or being put on a strict diet. Instead, your dietitian will aim to help you to develop an eating and activity plan to suit your needs and lifestyle and to work with you to set realistic and achievable goals. And these goals are not just about weight—having more energy, improving insulin levels, and regulating your periods are just some of the goals you might want to work on with the help of your dietitian. There is no need to worry about being judged by the scales—in fact many dietitians won't weigh you unless this is something that is important to you.

Registered Dietitians (RD) have a four-year college education, receive a Bachelor's Degree in Nutrition, complete an approved and accredited Dietetic Internship, and must pass a state board examination given by the Commission on Dietetic Registration (CDR) in order to become registered to practice dietetics. They are experts in the field of nutrition and have the knowledge, understanding, and clinical training to advise you on the best eating plan to meet your individual needs.

Your first consultation with a dietitian will generally take about an hour and will begin with collecting personal details, weight history, medical history, usual eating patterns and activity levels, and your goals and expectations for your consultations. This information will allow the dietitian to assess your needs and to provide information and education relevant to your situation.

The dietitian will then assist you in developing an eating plan to meet your individual needs as well as the information and ideas you need to put this into practice. The dietitian will generally want to see you again after a few weeks to review your progress and to provide further education as well as answer any questions you may have. How often you see the dietitian will be up to you—some people like to go along every week or two until they achieve their goals, while others only want one or two sessions to obtain the information they need.

To find a dietitian in your area see page 35.

Eating well

If you have PCOS, eating well is not just about managing your weight. Eating well can improve your overall health and energy levels, and can help to reduce your risk of heart disease and diabetes. It also means enjoying what you eat. The other thing to remember is that you need to eat in a way that helps to control your insulin levels. This means eating small regular meals and snacks spread across the day and choosing mostly healthy low-GI foods. Your healthy low-GI eating plan should include the following foods each day:

- fresh vegetables and salads
- fresh fruit
- whole-grain breads and cereals
- low-fat dairy products or non-dairy alternatives such as soy
- fish, lean meat, chicken, eggs, legumes, and soy products
- small amounts of healthy fats including nuts, seeds, avocado, olives, olive oil, canola oil, or peanut oil

We hope you have noticed that we are not asking you to remove a single food group. Cutting out certain sorts of foods is not a long-term solution, nor one that is good for your health or energy levels. Eating the healthy low-GI way is about choosing the right foods within *all* the food groups. For most women we see, it simply means swapping one food for another. There's always a tasty substitute. Trust us, we know plenty of them (see page 107).

Remember that when it comes to changing the way we eat, some people find this easy, but for the majority of us, change of any kind is difficult. Unlike altering bad habits such as smoking, changing the food we eat is rarely just a matter of giving up certain foods. A healthy diet contains a wide range of foods, but we need to eat them in the right amounts. The decisions behind what we eat are many and complex, and often some professional advice can help you to make the necessary changes. Helping people improve their diet is what dietitians do every day, so don't be shy. Give a dietitian a call if you need some help to get started. (See "How to Find a Dietitian" on page 35 to find a dietitian).

How do I change my diet?

Aim to make changes gradually.

Major changes to your diet, for example following a fad diet from a magazine article or current bestseller, are usually short-lived. Identify one aspect of your diet that you want to work on (for example, eating more vegetables) and make that your initial focus.

Attempt the easiest changes first.

Nothing inspires like success, so increase your chances by attacking the easiest changes first. For example, plan to eat one fruit snack each day.

Break big goals into a number of smaller, more achievable goals.

A big goal may be wanting to lose weight. This is unlikely to happen quickly, but it is attainable through gradual, consistent change. Smaller goals could be to exercise for 30 minutes every day and to reduce the saturated-fat content of your diet. Even smaller goals (which are the best way to begin) could be to do a 15-minute walk on alternate days and limit fast food meals to once a week.

Be prepared for setbacks.

It is normal to experience setbacks when making any type of change and lifestyle changes are no exception. If you find yourself getting off track, don't see this as a failure but as a natural stage in the progression to new habits. Remember, it usually takes about three months for a new change to become a habit. Accept lapses for what they are—you're only human—and get back on track the next day.

 Don't try to change everything overnight—start with a few small changes and add more as you achieve these.

4

Get Active with PCOS

REGULAR ACTIVITY AND EXERCISE are an essential part of managing PCOS. But when we talk about getting active, we don't just mean sweating it out at the gym. While regular planned exercise that gets your heart pumping and your muscles working is important, there is more to it than that. Being active when you have PCOS also means sitting less and moving more. You may not think that these things could make a difference, but they do!

> I was referred to a dietitian by my endocrinologist after being diagnosed with PCOS and insulin resistance. I had a history of heavy, really painful periods, mood swings, bloating, scalp hair loss, difficulties controlling my weight, and had been unable to fall pregnant despite trying IVF. At my first meeting I was wearing a size 18–22, and when asked, all I could say was that I wanted to be size 12 again. I had tried so many diets with no long-term success. The dietitian told me about healthy low-GI eating and gave me lots of ideas to improve my current eating habits to reduce fat and incorporate more healthy low-GI foods into my meals and snacks. It all sounded very achievable and I was confident that I could fit in a 20–30 minute walk most days. My endocrinologist started

*me on metformin at this point too. I saw the dietitian every month, and
each time I felt I was making positive changes to my diet and gradually
increasing my activity levels. I built up to walking an hour most morn-
ings as well as starting a strength training program at home on alternate
days. Most of all I made sure that I ate regularly, including lots of fruit
and vegetables, eating more fish and nuts, and switching most of my carbohydrate foods to low-GI choices. My energy levels improved significantly, and after ten months I was a size 14–16! And that was pretty
exciting. But even more exciting was the fact that at last I was pregnant!
I had a really easy pregnancy—mind you, I stuck carefully to my low-GI
eating plan and I exercised regularly right up until the birth. The good
news was that my blood glucose levels remained well controlled with no
signs of gestational diabetes. And as this book was being written, I gave
birth to a healthy baby girl.*
    Lisa, 32

Why exercise matters

Regular exercise is important for everyone, but particularly if you
have PCOS. Why?

- Exercise and activity speed up your metabolic rate (increasing the amount of energy you use), which helps you to balance your food intake and control your weight.
- Exercise and activity make your muscles more sensitive to insulin, which increases the amount of fat you burn.
- Exercise and activity help to reduce your risk of long-term
  health problems such as diabetes and heart disease. Research
  has shown that people who exercise regularly, even if they are
  overweight or have a family history of diabetes, have significantly less risk of developing diabetes.

Regular exercise has also been shown to:
- strengthen bones and muscles
- decrease anxiety and depression
- improve general well-being and quality of life

- improve blood fats
- reduce blood pressure
- improve strength and flexibility
- reduce body fat and increase lean body mass
- improve physical fitness
- enhance self-esteem and psychological well-being

If this isn't enough to convince you to get moving, a final but very important benefit of exercise is that it can help to reduce the loss of muscle that usually occurs with weight loss. When you lose weight through diet alone, you don't just lose fat but also a proportion of muscle. This isn't good, as a reduction in lean muscle mass means a reduction in your metabolism, which makes continued weight loss and maintaining your new weight more difficult. The good news is that including exercise as part of your weight loss plan can help to minimize this loss of muscle and maximize fat loss. One study in women with PCOS comparing diet only versus diet plus exercise (either aerobic or combined aerobic-resistance training) over 20 weeks found that while all groups lost similar amounts of weight, almost 50 percent of the weight loss in the diet-only group was due to a reduction in fat-free mass (i.e., muscle). The exercising groups lost approximately 45 percent more fat mass and 60 percent less fat-free mass than the diet-only group.

What type of exercise and how much?

Ideally you should try to fit in some activity on most days. Research has shown that just 30 minutes of moderate intensity exercise each day can help to improve your health, in particular reducing your risk of heart disease and diabetes. If you prefer, you can break this 30 minutes down to two sessions of 15 minutes or even three sessions of 10 minutes each and you will still see benefits.

If you are trying to lose weight, the more exercise you can do the better. In fact, the latest guidelines from the *American College of Sports Medicine* suggest that to prevent weight gain, we need to be exercising for 150 to 250 minutes per week, and to lose weight and keep it off we should be physically active for at least 250 minutes per week (that's roughly 1 hour on five days of the week or 40 minutes every day). Start with 30 minutes each day and build it up. If you can manage to be active for an hour most days you will certainly see the benefits. If you can't fit this in, do whatever you can—remember every little bit counts!

While aerobic exercise is generally thought of as the most effective for "fat-burning," and is certainly important, combining aerobic exercise with resistance training will give you even better results. Resistance training (also called strength training or weight training) helps to build muscle and increases your metabolism, assisting with weight loss. Research has also shown the benefits of resistance training for improving insulin resistance, reducing cardiovascular risk factors and improving blood glucose control in people with diabetes. And a number of studies have found that a combined aerobic and resistance training program is the best way to improve insulin resistance.

Resistance training: not just for the guys

Many women are scared of lifting weights as they think they will "bulk up," but this is unlikely unless you have a particularly muscular body type and are lifting really heavy weights. What weights can do is help you to become more toned, increase your metabolism, improve your body's sensitivity to insulin, and strengthen your bones.

You don't need to go to the gym to lift weights—with some basic equipment such as some hand weights, a resistance band, and a Swiss ball, you can easily do this at home. You can even use your own body weight for many exercises (think push-ups, chair squats, or triceps dips on the edge of a chair or low table). It is a good idea to get some instruction to begin with, to make sure you are doing the right exercises and doing them correctly (you don't want any injuries!). You could do this by organizing a few sessions with an exercise physiologist or personal trainer. There are also books and DVDs available; we recommend the Strong Women books and DVDs available at www.strongwomen.com/books. Developed by Dr. Miriam Nelson, these are written specifically for women and include easy-to-follow strength-training programs for home as well as a guide to exercises you can do at the gym.

A basic strength training program should include exercises for each of your main muscle groups (such as back, chest, legs, arms, and shoulders) and would normally include 2–3 sets of 8–12 repetitions of each exercise. This means that for each exercise you would lift the weight 8–12 times (more for lighter weights, and reducing the number of reps as you lift heavier weights) and then take a rest and repeat this another 1–2 times. You would then move on to the next exercise and do the same thing. You may do all the exercises each time you do your weights program or you could break it up and do, for example, upper body exercises on one day and lower body exercises on another day.

Interval training: getting the most out of your sessions

When it comes to aerobic exercise (the type that gets your heart pumping), there are many different options. But regardless of the type of exercise you do, if you want to make the most out of your exercise sessions, you should consider interval training. This means that throughout your exercise session you alternate between intervals of low to moderate intensity (a comfortable pace) and high intensity (a pace you can only sustain for a short period of time). The intensity of the exercise can be increased by going at a faster pace or by making the exercise more difficult. For example, if you were walking on a treadmill, you could increase the incline or add a jog for short periods of time, on an exercise bike you could up the speed or add more resistance. If you were walking outside you could pick a route with lots of hills or you could walk between one set of telegraph poles and sprint between the next set. You can start with very short high-intensity intervals every few minutes and gradually increase these or make them closer together as you get fitter. Research has shown that exercising in this way, rather than at a steady state, results in more fat loss, particularly around the middle, and greater improvements in insulin levels. It also makes your exercise sessions more interesting!

The final thing to remember is that variety is also important: the body becomes efficient at anything it does repeatedly, so after a while you'll stop seeing the results you initially got by doing what you are doing now. This is the time to add something new to your exercise program!

Our top ten ways to get moving

There are lots of options when it comes to being more active. The key is to find some activities that you enjoy. If exercise is a chore and you struggle to do it every day, it will be too hard to keep up.

Below are ten ideas to get you moving. You don't have to go solo. Exercising with friends is good for one and all. If you have had an injury of any sort, check it out with your doctor before you start any exercise program.

Walking

This is one of the best ways to get active, as it is easy, you can do it almost anywhere, and all you need to get started is a good pair of shoes. You don't have to climb a mountain, and it doesn't have to be a hike or a bushwalk. Simply start the day by walking to work or, if you are not a morning person, try walking home and arrive home stress free! If you don't like walking alone, grab a partner or friend and combine your workout with catching up on the day's news.

You could also get off the bus or train a stop or two earlier and walk the rest of the way, or fit in a walk at lunchtime for a chance to stretch and get some fresh air. On the weekend, consider a longer walk at the beach or park or try hiking or mountain climbing. You could also fit more walking into your day by walking short distances instead of taking the car; walking the kids to school or taking them for a walk to the park; taking the dog for a walk around the block; or catching up with a friend for a walk on the beach rather than a coffee.

If you are not sure whether walking is really effective, then consider this: a recent study that followed a large group of young adults over a 15-year period found a significant association between walking and annual weight gain, particularly for those who were heavier. For example, in women at the 75th percentile for baseline weight (meaning they were heavier than 75 percent of other study participants when the study began), walking for 30 minutes per day resulted in

17-pound less weight gain over 15 years compared to women who did no leisure-time walking.

Dancing

Dancing is a lot of fun as well as being a great way to get your blood pumping. There are a variety of classes available, either through community centers or privately, including ballroom, ballet, funk, jazz, Latin, tango, hip hop, and belly dancing. You don't have to know how—find a beginners' class and go along for some fun. Most teachers will tell you that if you can walk you can dance! If you are not brave enough to join a class, or don't have time, clear some room at home, turn your favorite music up loud and start grooving!

Treadmills and exercise bikes

If time is an issue or you are not an outdoors sort of person these are an ideal option. Buy or rent a treadmill or bike for home and you can use it whenever it suits you—without worrying about the weather. You can also save time by combining your exercise with reading (for work or pleasure) or watching your favorite TV show. Otherwise listening to some good music will ensure you keep your heart rate up and will make the time go faster.

Exercise classes

Fitness centers, community centers, and private studios all run a variety of classes such as aerobics, step, kickboxing, yoga, and Pilates. If you are not sure about joining a class, or you can't find one to fit your time schedule, you can buy exercise DVDs to use at home or try renting one from your local DVD store or library.

Play a sport

Basketball, soccer, touch football, tennis, or golf to name just a few—why not join a local competition or organize a game with friends?

Swimming and aqua-aerobics

If you like the water, these may be the best exercises for you. Water exercises are also particularly good for anyone with joint problems as your weight is supported in the water. Head to your favorite pool and see what they have to offer. Aqua-aerobic classes are also held at many fitness centers and hospitals.

Cycling

Cycling is not only a great way to get fit but it can also be a cheap means of commuting (which is also great for the environment). If time is your biggest barrier to a fitness program, cycling may also be a way of turning your daily travel into exercise without finding extra time in the day. For those who don't like cycling outdoors, an indoor cycle can turn television watching into exercise time. Most gyms and health clubs offer indoor cycling classing (spinning) as well as machines for individualized workouts.

Rowing

Outdoor or indoor, rowing is a great all-over workout that will have you fit in no time! If you can't see yourself getting out on the water in a rowboat, canoe, or kayak, the next best thing is to buy or rent a rowing machine for home or use one at your local fitness center.

Household chores

Master the art of getting two jobs done at once—your exercise and your household chores. You may not think of these activities as exercise, but cleaning, dusting, vacuuming, and mopping will all give you a good workout as will washing the car, mowing the lawn, sweeping, and digging in the garden. Put on your favorite music while you work and put in your best effort—you won't only get a great workout but you will have the reward of a clean house, shiny car, or neat and tidy yard at the end.

A few more ideas . . .

In-line skating, ice skating, jumping rope, cycling—the possibilities are endless! Pick the activity that you think you will enjoy most and get moving!

Building more activity into your day

Sitting less

Recent research had found that regardless of whether or not you are a regular exerciser, the amount of time you spend sitting can have a big impact on your health. That's right—even if you get out for a walk or to the gym each morning but you spend the rest of your day sitting at a computer and your evenings in front of the television, your risk of metabolic problems like insulin resistance, diabetes, and heart disease increase. In fact, one study found that sedentary time was a better predictor of insulin resistance than aerobic fitness or time spent in physical activity. And a number of studies have linked television watching with an increased risk of diabetes and metabolic syndrome. One study found that women who watched 14 hours of television or more per week had a 50 percent increased risk of abnormal glucose tolerance (either prediabetes or type 2 diabetes).

What does all of this mean? Building a regular exercise habit is essential, but it is also important to find ways to spend less time being inactive. Here are a few tips for sitting less:

- Regularly get up from your desk to stretch or take a quick walk around the office or outside
- Walk to talk to a colleague rather than using the phone or e-mail
- Do household chores or a few exercises during television ad breaks
- Have a "walking meeting" with work colleagues
- Stand while talking on the phone
- Limit television viewing to no more than two hours per day

Moving more

In addition to planned exercise, just moving more throughout the day can make a big difference. Cars, computers, dishwashers, washing machines, cell phones, and e-mail mean that many of us get very little activity in our day. Remember, becoming more active means thinking about exercise or movement as an opportunity, not an inconvenience. Consider the ways you could get a little more movement in your day—every little bit counts!

- Take the stairs instead of the elevator. Make this a policy!
- Wash the car by hand rather than going to the car wash. Put the money you save toward a reward for yourself.
- Walk to get the weekend papers rather than getting them delivered. You will feel like you have earned the right to sit in the sun and read when you get back.
- Park a little farther from the shops rather than looking for the closest spot. This will also save the time and frustration of driving around in circles looking for that spot you can never find.
- Walk short distances rather than taking the car. This also saves on gas and you will be doing your part for the environment.
- Get off the train or bus a few stops earlier and walk the rest of the way.
- Walk the kids to school rather than driving them.
- Walk or cycle to work. One study found that so-called active commuters' were 50 percent less likely to be obese and had lower levels of blood fats, insulin levels, and blood pressure.

Research has shown that we need to take about 7,500 steps each day to maintain weight and 10,000 steps to lose weight. If you want to see how much you move (or don't move!), buy a pedometer (step-counter) and see how far you go. A pedometer can be a good motivator to moving more. They are available from most sports shops. It's both fun and a challenge. Give it a try!

Remember: every little bit counts.

In summary

There are lots of ways to get active if you have PCOS—do all of them and you will get the best results:

1. Sit less. Work out ways you can spend less time being inactive.
2. Move more. Find a few ways to build more incidental activity into your day.
3. Exercise most days. Aim for at least 40 minutes but up to 1 hour for the best results when it comes to losing weight and keeping it off.

4. Add intervals. Once you are exercising regularly, add some high-intensity intervals to your workout to fast-track your fat loss and really improve insulin resistance.

5. Lift weights. Whether at the gym or at home, aim for 2–3 sessions per week of resistance training, to build muscle, improve your metabolism, and improve how insulin works in your body.

How to stay motivated? That's not just *your* problem

Many of the women who talk to us say that they find it difficult to get started with exercise and even more challenging to continue a regular exercise program. If this sounds like you, you are not alone! Research has shown that of all those who start an exercise program, only about a third continue with it beyond three months. To increase your chance of success, it is important to think about the things that may help motivate you to start and continue exercising. Here are some pointers that have helped the women we see to get started and to keep going with their exercise programs:

Women who get active and stay active:

1. Set realistic short-term and long-term goals.
2. Understand the benefits that exercise will provide.
3. Start slowly and gradually increase what they do as it gets easier.
4. Include a variety of activities that are enjoyable and fun.
5. Choose times and locations that are convenient.
6. Make sure their exercise program is flexible and fits in with their lifestyle.
7. Monitor and reward their progress.
8. Exercise with others—make a commitment to them.
9. Think of exercise as an investment of their time (and a good one at that!) rather than something that takes time.
10. Recognize the rewards exercise is providing, even when the weight isn't dropping off—exercise improves your sensitivity to insulin regardless of weight loss as well as increasing fitness, strength, and energy levels.

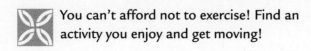 You can't afford not to exercise! Find an activity you enjoy and get moving!

5

Take Care of Yourself

EATING WELL AND BEING ACTIVE are the cornerstones of managing PCOS, but there are a few other things that you can do to help yourself that are very important for improving your overall health, energy levels, and feeling of well-being.

Taking care of yourself is essential and what we call the four Ss make up the final part of your four-step plan. This means:

- surviving stress
- sleeping soundly
- seeking support
- stopping smoking

Surviving stress

This really is the S word isn't it? Stress is a part of life for most of us and can't be avoided. While you may be able to eliminate some of the stress in your life, the key to managing stress effectively is to increase your ability to cope with the stresses and strains you face.

The additional problem with stress for women with PCOS is that it can upset hormonal balance, increase blood glucose levels, blood fats and blood pressure, reduce immunity, and upset digestion. A recent study found that women who experienced high stress levels at work had double the risk of developing type 2 diabetes. Stress also sends many of us heading straight for the fridge door!

Unfortunately, PCOS itself tends to create extra stress. First you must you deal with the physical symptoms—excess hair, skin problems, managing weight, and, for some, being unable to become pregnant.

Then there are the emotional consequences of living with PCOS—an often forgotten part of dealing with this condition. Having PCOS can impact significantly on body image and self-esteem and this, in turn, can affect your ability to cope with the problems you face. Enhancing self-esteem and improving body image are an important part of your PCOS management plan.

Remember that it is absolutely normal at some stage to feel fed up, frustrated, or overwhelmed by PCOS. At the same time, it is really important to know that it is completely reasonable and understandable to feel like this and it's okay to seek help. If you feel unable to cope on your own you should seek some professional help—find a psychologist or counselor who can help you to deal with the issues you face.

PCOS impacts health-related quality of life— it's not all in your head

A number of studies have found that the symptoms typically associated with PCOS, including changes in physical appearance, menstrual disturbances, and infertility, result in psychological distress and a reduced quality of life. A large recent study comparing women with PCOS and those without PCOS found that more than two-thirds of women with PCOS were classified as depressed while another identified psychological problems in 62 percent of women with PCOS compared with 26 percent in a similar group of women without PCOS. Furthermore, PCOS has been found to impact negatively on psychological Health-Related Quality of Life (HRQoL), even when compared with other serious health conditions such as diabetes, coronary heart disease, epilepsy, and arthritis.

My doctor referred me to an endocrinologist because I was always tired, gaining weight, and had terrible mood swings. After tests it became clear that my routine blood and thyroid function tests were absolutely normal but I had a slight enlargement of the thyroid. We decided to wait and see . . . and I made an appointment for a follow-up review three months later. By the time the review happened, I had gained 6½ pounds, and my constant fatigue and mood swings were interfering with my effectiveness as an executive and with my home life. By this time my endocrinologist suspected PCOS and, on questioning, I realized that my periods were two to three days longer than they had been six months earlier. I also remembered that my hairdresser had commented that the hair on the top of my head was thinning. The endocrinologist also noticed that there was excess hair around my right nipple and naval line. Tests showed that my serum LH was markedly elevated. That's when I was scheduled an internal ultrasound, which showed unequivocal evidence of PCOS. I was prescribed metformin, a healthy low-GI diet, and aerobic exercise. I lost around 33 pounds over a three-month period and started to feel much better about myself—I was even promoted at work! That's when I decided to do an MBA part-time to further my career, but it all became too much. I found it hard to meet all my deadlines and look after myself properly; I was always rushing. I was too busy to exercise, I ate whatever I could lay my hands on and, worst of all, I forgot to renew my prescription for metformin. It was also a very anxious time for the whole family as my mother was diagnosed with Alzheimer's. I missed two appointments at the clinic and when I finally went back and jumped on the scales I had put on 37 pounds. By this time my periods were irregular and I had dark coarse facial hair and acne. I went back on my program of healthy low-GI eating, exercise, and metformin. It wasn't easy, but I did get my MBA!

Christine, 28

How Do You Cope with Stress?

	Always	Sometimes	Never
Do you exercise regularly? Do you communicate feelings to others?			
Do you take time out for activities you enjoy?			
Do you remain positive and optimistic, even during difficult times?			
Do you practice any formal relaxation techniques such as meditation?			
Do you manage your time effectively and get all your important tasks done each day?			

Mostly "Always"

Congratulations—you should be able to cope well with the stress that life presents you. Managing stress has many important health benefits so keep up the good work!

Mostly "Sometimes"

You are halfway there but there is more you could be doing to cope with stress. Pick the areas you are not doing so well in and build in some strategies to help. For example, if you are stressed by your never-ending "to-do pile" and never seem to have time for yourself, start with learning to manage your time more effectively—write lists, prioritize, and schedule some relaxation time for yourself.

Mostly "Never"

It's likely that you are not coping well with the stress in your life and this could be impacting negatively on your health and well-being. There are many things you could do to increase your ability to deal with stress: starting a regular exercise program; taking some time out for activities you enjoy; and finding someone to talk to about your feelings would be a great start.

Thousands of people tend to turn to food when under pressure. If you are like them you need to find other ways of coping. It may seem a little like homework, but it's useful to write yourself a list of all those things you would like to do that you never get time to fit in—most of us have lots of these! This list can be a useful prompt, especially if you stick it on the fridge door!

Here are some ideas that many women with PCOS have told us that they find useful. These suggestions may help to get you started, but don't forget to add your own:

Read a good book
Take a bubble bath
Spend time in the garden
Write to a friend
Clean out your wardrobe
Have a massage
Go to bed early and read
Sit in the sun and read the paper
Redecorate your house
Listen to music
Watch a good movie
Give yourself a pedicure
Buy yourself some flowers
Get a haircut
Take a weekend away
Visit the zoo
Learn something new
Have a facial
Look at photographs
Go for a drive
Buy some new clothes

Sleeping soundly

Getting enough sleep is vital. A lack of sleep can have many negative consequences—reducing immunity, increasing the level of stress

Sleep Disturbance

It's not uncommon for women with PCOS to have difficulties sleeping, such as having trouble getting off to sleep or experiencing disrupted sleep. This may be due to hormonal fluctuations, particularly around the time of your periods, and may also be a result of stress. Carrying extra weight, particularly around the middle, can also lead to sleep disturbances including sleep apnea. This is a condition where breathing is disrupted during sleep due to blockages to the windpipe—symptoms include snoring and stopping breathing for short periods while asleep. Studies have shown that women with PCOS are up to 30 times more likely to suffer from sleep apnea than women without PCOS, and this appears to be more likely if you have insulin resistance, irrespective of your weight. If you suffer from any form of sleep disturbance on an ongoing basis (or your partner tells you that you snore!), you should seek professional help. Poor sleep can lead to excessive daytime sleepiness and will reduce energy levels, increase stress, and make exercise more difficult. And sleep apnea is a serious condition that, if left untreated, can lead to other health problems such as high blood pressure and diabetes.

hormones, and worsening insulin resistance. In fact a number of studies in healthy subjects have shown that sleep deprivation leads to a significant worsening of insulin sensitivity, even over short periods of time. Research has also linked poor sleep (generally less than six hours per night) with diabetes risk; in one study, those who slept for less than five hours per night were three times more likely to develop diabetes; other studies have shown a 10–50 percent increased risk for those sleeping five to six hours per night. Being tired also worsens memory, reduces productivity, and makes it harder to get enthusiastic about exercising and eating well. Finally, lack of sleep can make it harder to cope with stress.

If you're not getting enough sleep, you're not alone. While most adults need at least eight hours sleep, statistics show that a large proportion of the population sleep for seven hours or less each night. Most adults also report difficulties sleeping at some time.

Our message to you is that sleep is just as important as diet and exercise. Make an effort to get your eight hours and if you have difficulties sleeping, try the tips below or seek some professional help.

Tips for getting a good night's sleep:

- Exercise regularly but avoid strenuous exercise close to bedtime.
- Go to bed and get up at the same time each day (+/- an hour on Sunday!).
- Get some bright light (preferably outdoors) first thing in the morning and avoid bright lights at night. Use dimmers or lamps in the evening and eat dinner by candlelight; this can help with your body's sleep-wake cycle.
- Relax for an hour before bed—avoid stimulating activities such as scary movies and loud music.
- Try not to work right up to bedtime and make sure you finish your workday by writing down a list of things you need to do tomorrow so that your brain doesn't work hard to remember them all night.
- Make sure your bedroom is quiet, dark, and a comfortable temperature before you go to bed—noise, light, and being too hot or cold will all make it harder to get a good night's sleep.
- If you have trouble getting to sleep, get up and read for twenty minutes, try a glass of warm milk, or listen to a relaxation tape. Research has shown that they do work.
- Try a glass of warm milk or an herbal tea such as chamomile or valerian before bed.
- Lavender essential oil has been shown to help with sleep—try burning some in an oil burner or sprinkle a few drops on your pillow.

Seeking support

Having a good support team can make all the difference when you have PCOS. Many of the women we see comment on the fact that they feel very much alone in living with their condition and feel that

PCOS and Complementary and Alternative Medicine

Complementary therapies include herbal medicine, nutrition, acupuncture, homeopathy, osteopathy, chiropractic, traditional Chinese medicine, aromatherapy, reflexology, and remedial therapy such as massage and kinesiology.

There have been a small number of studies performed on the effects of Chinese herbal medicine or herbal supplements on reproductive symptoms (fertility, ovulation, etc.) and insulin resistance in PCOS. In these studies, the alternative therapy often has not been compared directly to the effect of a standard treatment (lifestyle or medical), so it is difficult to say how effective these treatments are. As yet, the results are preliminary, but larger, controlled clinical studies are needed before any comment on their usefulness, either in combination with current therapy or instead of current therapy, is made.

Natural remedies should only be prescribed by an experienced qualified practitioner—preferably with an interest in women's health and PCOS. Your general practitioner or specialist should be informed about all natural remedies you are taking.

Source: www.managingpcos.org.au.

no one else understands what they are going through. Talking about these feelings and meeting other women in the same boat can be a big help.

The good news is that there *is* support out there for women with PCOS. From formal PCOS support groups to understanding health professionals you can find the care and attention that you need.

Your team of health professionals might include a GP, endocrinologist, gynecologist, and dietitian. You may also want to seek the help of a psychologist, exercise physiologist, or personal trainer and natural health practitioner. PCOS support groups can provide you with valuable information and contact with others through meetings, newsletters, Web sites, and e-mail discussion groups.

You could also seek out other groups such as infertility support groups. Ask your health professional for a referral or look in the *Yellow Pages* for contact details.

About PCOS Support Groups

PCOS support groups provide information, education, and support to women with PCOS as well as their partners, family, and friends. From face-to-face meetings and e-mail chat groups to newsletters and Web sites, they provide the opportunity for women to come together for mutual support and friendship and provide the information to empower women with PCOS to take charge of their condition. Many of these groups also work hard to raise the public awareness of PCOS and the effects it has on the lives of so many women, and encourage research that could lead to a cure or more effective treatment. The details for support groups are included in the back of this book—we encourage you to contact them and find out how you can get involved.

Stopping smoking

If you smoke, giving up smoking is one of the most important things you can do to improve your health and the health of those around you. Everyone these days is well aware that smoking increases the risk of heart disease and cancer. Did you also know that smoking worsens insulin sensitivity and reduces fertility? Or that heavy smokers (20 or more per day) are 60 percent more likely to develop diabetes? All smokers with PCOS should quit, and this is particularly important if you are trying to fall pregnant.

Quitting smoking is not easy, so if you have made the decision to quit but need some help in doing so, talk to your doctor or health care professional, call your local or state health department for assistance with a toll-free Quit Line, or visit the Office of the Surgeon General's Tobacco Cessation Guideline Web site at www.surgeon-general.gov/tobacco. The American Cancer Society, sponsors of the annual "Great American Smokeout," also offers useful information online at www.cancer.org.

 Take time out to take care of yourself. Reducing and managing stress and getting enough sleep will give you the time and energy to focus on making other lifestyle changes. Seek support if you need to. If you are a smoker, stop now!

6

Putting the GI to Work in Your Day

THIS CHAPTER LAYS OUT the practical part of the low-GI lifestyle and explains how to make the change to the healthy low-GI way of eating.

Remember that eating the healthy low-GI way is not a diet. It means changing your eating habits in a way that will last you a lifetime. It's not about weighing, counting, or measuring and it's not about eating foods you dislike or cutting out the foods you enjoy most. What it is about is eating the right foods—the foods that fill you up, give you more energy, and improve your health and, best of all, your PCOS symptoms.

There are plenty of choices when it comes to healthy low-GI eating, which is why the women we see comment that this is the easiest "diet" they have ever followed. They don't feel hungry; they can still eat foods they enjoy; they have more energy and their cravings subside. In essence, they feel good and their new way of eating feels sustainable. And if it's sustainable it's likely to work.

I understand GI but what is GL and what does it mean?

It is important to consider both the GI of the food and the amount of carbohydrate it contains—that is, the total glycemic load; this is a true measure of the effect of your meal or snack on your blood glucose and insulin levels. You can calculate the glycemic load (GL) by multiplying the GI by the amount of carbohydrate per serving and then dividing by 100. For example, 1 cup of watermelon has a GI of 72 and a carbohydrate content of 10g, giving a GL of 7, while a medium apple has a GI of 38 and a carbohydrate content of 15g, giving a GL of 6. So although watermelon has a higher GI than other fruits, its high water content means that eaten in moderate amounts, it is comparable to other fruits with a lower GI. GL tells us that small amounts of a high-GI food are unlikely to have a big impact on blood glucose and insulin levels while large servings of a low-GI food can still raise blood glucose and insulin levels significantly. It's best to aim for foods that have a GL less than 10 with the total for the whole day less than 100. In summary, consider the amount you are eating as well as the GI of the food! Our menus and recipes are designed to take into account both GI and GL.

The optimum diet for women with PCOS

The optimum diet for women with PCOS is one that is low in saturated fat and contains moderate amounts of protein and carbohydrate, with most of the carbohydrate choices being low GI. It should contain plenty of vegetables, salads, fruit, legumes, and whole grains.

This type of eating plan will help achieve weight management, boost energy levels, improve insulin sensitivity, and reduce the risk of health problems such as diabetes and heart disease.

To make it easy for you we have developed seven dietary guidelines. These aren't rules; they are a simple guide to inspire you to improve your eating habits for life. Then, to help you to implement these guidelines, we explain in detail how you can translate them into daily meals and snacks. Finally we finish this section with a shopping list and sample meal plans to get you started.

Seven dietary guidelines for women with PCOS

1. Eat seven or more servings of vegetables and fruit each day.
2. Choose whole-grain breads and cereals with a low GI.
3. Eat more legumes (dried beans, peas, and lentils).
4. Include nuts in your diet regularly.

5. Eat more fish and seafood, particularly oily fish like salmon and sardines.
6. Choose lean meats and low-fat dairy products.
7. Choose monounsaturated and omega-3 polyunsaturated fats such as olive and canola oil, fish, nuts, seeds, and avocado.

Low GI or Low Carb

When you have PCOS, reducing insulin levels is important. When it comes to the food you eat, the key to reducing insulin levels is reducing the glycemic load (GL) of your diet. There are two ways to do this—reduce the GI of your diet overall or reduce your carbohydrate intake. Many of the women we see try the second option first because it sounds easy to cut carbohydrate foods out of their diet. While this may help short term, it is not the answer for long-term good health and management of your PCOS.

The reason for this is that low-carbohydrate diets can worsen insulin resistance and they eliminate many of the foods we know are important for good health and reducing risk of diseases such as cancer, heart disease, and type 2 diabetes. Low-carbohydrate diets also tend to lower energy levels, making exercise more difficult. A diet based on low-GI foods, on the other hand, gives you the best of both worlds—enough carbohydrates for optimum insulin sensitivity, nutrition, and energy levels without an excessive GL.

If weight loss is a goal, high-carbohydrate diets are probably not the answer for you either—as with most things, moderation is the key. Whether you have a high or moderate carbohydrate intake, however, you should choose mostly healthy low-GI carbs.

The good news is that eating the low-GI way will mean that you feel fuller and will be less likely to overeat. This means that measuring, counting, and weighing your food can be a thing of the past. You will also find that when you are choosy about your carbohydrates, your insulin levels will be lower and you will therefore burn more fat. Over time, and combined with some regular exercise, this will result in weight loss.

I have asthma and over a very wheezy six-month period I had to have two back-to-back courses of high-dose steroids by mouth (as well as antibiotics). That's when I put on 22 pounds predominantly around my middle and upper thighs. Despite working out in the gym doing aerobic exercises 3–4 times a week and going on what I thought was a weight-reducing diet I was absolutely unable to shed any of the weight I had put on during the steroid treatment. So I went to see my doctor, who sent me off to an endocrinologist. All the tests he did seemed absolutely normal. However, he did say that I might be insulin resistant and recommended a healthy low-GI diet that I followed religiously—and in the first ten days lost 5½ pounds. It's such an easy diet to follow, I recommended it to many of my friends and to my daughter.

Didi, 56

1. Eat seven or more servings of vegetables and fruit every day

Fruit and vegetables should form a major part of any healthy eating plan. They are rich sources of vitamins, minerals, antioxidants, and phytochemicals, all of which are important for good health and can help to protect you against diseases such as cancer and cardiovascular disease. They are also high in fiber, helping to fill you up and, apart from avocado and olives that contain "healthy" monounsaturated fats, fruits and vegetables are very low in fat.

Apart from the starchy vegetables: potato, sweet potato, corn, and yam, most vegetables have very little carbohydrate so do not have a GI value. Potatoes generally have a high GI, while sweet potato, corn, and yam have a relatively low GI. This means that if you are a big potato eater, you should try to replace some potato for these lower GI starchy vegetables. And when you do choose potato, try to go for the baby new potatoes, which have a lower GI than other varieties. Vegetables like pumpkin and carrot have a GI value but there is very little carbohydrate in a normal serving of these vegetables so we suggest that you consider them as "free foods." All green vegetables and salad vegetables can also be eaten freely and you should aim to eat at least five servings of vegetables each day—one serving is half a cup of cooked vegetables or one cup of salad vegetables.

When choosing vegetables, variety is the key—don't just stick with the same old varieties like beans, carrots, and peas. Spinach, bok choy, broccoli, cauliflower, cabbage, Brussels sprouts, peppers, tomato, cucumber, arugula, asparagus, zucchini, snow peas, and eggplant—the possibilities are endless. Why not buy something different each time you shop? Aim to make your plate as colorful as possible. Ask your grocer what's in season right now.

All fruits contain carbohydrate from their natural sugar content. Most fruits have a low or moderate GI, with the exception of watermelon, which has a high GI. This doesn't mean you need to avoid higher GI fruits like melons—these fruits have a lower carbohydrate intake due to the amount of water they contain so their GL, or overall effect on blood glucose and insulin levels, is still relatively small. In general, temperate fruits like apples and pears tend to have a lower GI and tropical fruits like melons and pineapple tend to have a moderate to high GI. Try to include a variety of fruit as part of your low-GI eating plan and aim for at least two servings each day—one serving is a medium piece like an apple or banana or 2–3 smaller pieces like plums and apricots.

Use the following ideas to get your seven servings each day:

Breakfast

- Include fruit (fresh, canned in natural juice, or dried) with your breakfast cereal.
- Try a fresh fruit smoothie for a quick but satisfying breakfast meal.
- For a more substantial breakfast, add some vegetables on your toast—try asparagus, mushrooms, tomato, and onion or sliced tomato and avocado.
- Mushrooms, asparagus, and tomato are also good added to omelets.

Lunch

- Add plenty of salad vegetables on your sandwich—try tomato, lettuce, cucumber, sprouts, beets, grated carrot, and strips of red, green, or yellow peppers.
- For toasted sandwiches go for tomato, roasted sweet pepper, mushroom, sweet potato, olives, zucchini and eggplant.
- Use avocado as a spread on your sandwich instead of butter.
- Salads are a great way to fill up at lunchtime and the possibilities are endless—don't stick with lettuce, tomato, and cucumber, try adding snow peas, hot chili peppers, corn, green beans, steamed broccoli, asparagus, roasted sweet potato and eggplant, sun-dried tomatoes, and a few cubes of avocado or some olives.
- For colder weather, soups are a great way to get more vegetables into your diet—try pumpkin, sweet potato, lentil, split pea, minestrone, or tomato.

Dinner

- Include vegetables or salads with all main meals—serve them steamed, seasoned with fresh or dried herbs, or with a dressing made from olive oil, lemon juice, balsamic vinegar, and garlic.
- Always have some frozen vegetables handy for when you haven't had time to shop for fresh varieties.
- If you don't like vegetables on their own, add them to stir-fries, curries, casseroles, and grated or chopped into meat dishes.
- Choose vegetable-based dishes when eating out or ask for a side salad with your meal.

Snacks and desserts

- Fruit and grated vegetables such as carrot and zucchini can be added into cakes and muffins.

- Choose fruit for snacks—fruit is widely available, inexpensive and easy to eat, without the added fat and sugar found in many other snack foods.
- Serve raw vegetables such as celery, carrot, cucumber, sweet peppers, broccoli, or cauliflower florets as a snack served with a low-fat dip or salsa.
- Make fruit the basis of your desserts—try baked apples, fruit crumbles, whole wheat filo with fruit, and canned fruit with low-fat custard, yogurt, or ice cream.

2. Eat whole-grain breads and cereals with a low glycemic index

Cereal grains including rice, wheat, oats, barley, quinoa, rye, and products made from them (including bread, pasta, breakfast cereal, and flours) are the most concentrated sources of carbohydrates that we eat, so have a major impact on the GI of our diet.

Whole-grain breads and cereals have many health benefits. Most have a lower glycemic index than refined cereal grains and they are also nutritionally superior, containing higher levels of fiber, vitamins, minerals, and phytochemicals. We know from studies that higher consumption of cereal fiber and whole grains is associated with a reduced incidence of type 2 diabetes, cancer, and heart disease.

Unfortunately, our Western diet tends to be based on highly processed grains and flours, which are quickly digested and result in a much greater rise in blood glucose and insulin levels than is desirable. Since high insulin levels are something you want to avoid when you have PCOS, substituting processed grains and cereals for those with a lower GI is a very important part of making the change to a healthy low-GI diet. Lower GI choices include oats, whole-grain and sourdough breads, bulgur, barley, most types of pasta and noodles, and longer grain varieties of rice such as basmati, Uncle Ben's converted, long-grain rice, and Uncle Ben's long-grain and wild rice blend.

To eat more breads and cereals with a low GI try the following ideas:

Breakfast

- Old-fashioned oatmeal is one of the best breakfast choices around—it's inexpensive, has no added fats or sugars and is really satisfying, particularly on a cold morning! Add some stewed apple, a few raisins, and a sprinkle of cinnamon for sweetness and top with low-fat milk or soy milk. Remember to choose the whole oats rather than the instant varieties, which have a much higher GI due to all that processing.
- In warmer weather choose cereals based on wheat bran, psyllium, and oats such as natural muesli and Kellogg's All-Bran.
- For those who prefer toast, choose whole-grain or sourdough bread or try a 9-grain English muffin.

Lunch

- For sandwiches, go for grainy breads made with barley, rye, flaxseed, triticale, sunflower seed, oats, soy, and cracked wheat. You could also try sourdough or pumpernickel breads.
- Barley can be added to soups to make a satisfying winter lunch.
- Pita bread also has a lower GI—try a pita filled with hummus and tabbouli (made from cracked wheat) or for colder weather a pita pizza topped with tomato, red pepper, mushrooms, avocado, a few olives, and a sprinkle of grated cheese.
- If you are buying lunch out, try a small pasta with tomato-based sauce, Asian noodle soups, or tandoori chicken with basmati rice.

Dinner

- Choose Asian noodles such as Hokkien, rice, or egg noodles in place of rice.
- Try low-GI rices such as basmati, Uncle Ben's converted, long grain rice, and Uncle Ben's long grain and wild rice blend.

- Barley can be added into soups and casseroles or used in place of rice—it has a nutty, chewy texture.
- Try quinoa in place of rice. It can be used in a similar way to couscous, in salads, or as a base to casseroles or stews.

Snacks and desserts

- Whole-grain fruit bread with ricotta makes a satisfying snack for those with a sweet tooth.
- Baked pita bread is a healthy alternative to chips, served with salsa or hummus.
- Try whole-grain crackers (e.g., Ryvita light rye whole-grain crispbread) topped with ricotta, avocado, or hummus and sliced tomato.
- For dessert you could try a fruit crumble with oat topping, creamed rice made with low-GI rice, or bread pudding made with whole-grain fruit bread.

3. Eat more legumes (beans, peas, and lentils)

For a low-GI food that's easy on the budget, versatile, filling, low in calories, and nutritious, look no further than legumes—that bag of dried kidney beans, or package of lentils or can of chickpeas in the kitchen cupboard! Whether you buy dried beans and cook them yourself at home, or opt for the very convenient, time-saving canned varieties, you are choosing one of nature's lowest GI foods.

Legumes are also high in fiber—both soluble and insoluble—and packed with nutrients providing a valuable source of protein, carbohydrate, B vitamins, folate, and minerals. Sprouted dried beans—such as mung, soy, chickpeas, and lentils—are excellent sources of vitamin C and are great eaten raw in a salad or stir-fried. Legumes are an important part of the healthy low-GI way of eating. Try to put them on the menu at least twice a week, more often if you are vegetarian. Legumes also make a great naturally gluten-free low-GI carb for those with celiac disease or gluten intolerance.

So, what are legumes? Legumes (also known as pulses) are the edible dried seeds found inside the mature pods of leguminous plants (e.g., beans, peas, and lentils). Nutritionally, they are quite different from fresh, young green beans and peas, which don't have as much protein or fiber because their water content is high.

Legumes can be bought either dried or canned. Canned legumes are ready to use (they only need heating through) and meals based on these are much faster to prepare than meat-based meals. Dried legumes need a little more preparation—most need to be soaked before cooking—but are worth the effort and can be frozen in small batches so they are ready to use at any time. Soaked or cooked beans can be kept in an airtight container for several days in the fridge. All legumes have a low GI, including dried and canned varieties, although the canned varieties are a little higher than those you cook yourself.

Thanks to a tendency to cause intestinal gas, legumes have generally had a bad name. But not all legumes will make you gassy, and not everyone has the problem. Cooking legumes thoroughly in fresh water (not in the water you soaked them in) and rinsing the canned varieties helps; as does eating them regularly—it can improve your tolerance.

Tofu (soy bean curd) is an easy way of using soy. It has a mild flavor itself but absorbs the flavors of other foods, making it delicious when it's been marinated in soy sauce, ginger, and garlic and tossed into a stir-fry. Tofu contains very little carbohydrate so doesn't have a GI value.

With such variety and versatility, incorporating legumes into your meals a few times a week is easy—here are some ideas to help you to make these "superfoods" a more regular part of your diet.

Breakfast

- Hummus on toast makes an easy and satisfying breakfast.
- Try scrambling silken tofu in place of eggs—add some fresh or dried herbs and chopped tomato and sauté in a little olive oil.

Lunch

- Lentil, split pea, or minestrone soup all make a satisfying winter lunch.
- Baked bean or black bean enchiladas—an easy all-time favorite!

- Add a can of three-bean mix or some chickpeas to create a salad that really fills you up.
- Lentils or chickpeas can be made into burgers and served on a roll or pita bread. If you don't have time to make your own burgers, pre-prepared varieties can be found in the chilled section of the supermarket. A great alternative for the barbecue.
- Spread hummus (made from chickpeas) on your sandwich in place of butter.

Dinner

- Add red kidney beans to ground meat to serve with tacos, burritos, pasta, or rice.
- Chickpeas have a nutty flavor and go well in curries and stir-fries.
- Make some dahl (lentils cooked with spices) as an accompaniment to your next curry.
- Green soy beans make a tasty addition to a stir-fry. They have a nutty texture and can be bought frozen in most Asian grocery stores.
- Add cannellini, borlotti, or black-eye peas (which are really beans) to stews and casseroles.
- Firm tofu can be cubed, marinated, and added into stir-fries or threaded onto skewers with vegetables to make kebabs for the barbecue or grill.
- Substitute lentils in place of meat in dishes such as shepherd's pie and lasagna.

Snacks and desserts

- Silken tofu can be used in place of cream cheese to make desserts such as cheesecake.
- Roasted chickpeas or soy beans make a tasty and satisfying snack.
- Try a small can of baked beans or four-bean mix for a snack if you are really hungry.
- For a healthy dip go for hummus or puree bean spread with carrot and celery sticks.

Cooking with Legumes

Dried legumes: dried beans and peas need soaking and cooking before you use them in your meals. Lentils and split peas cook much faster and don't need soaking.

- To *soak* beans, place them in a saucepan and cover with two to three times their volume of cold water—soak overnight or during the day. If time is limited, take a shortcut by adding three times the volume of water to rinsed beans, bringing to a boil for a few minutes then removing from heat and letting them soak for an hour.
- To *cook*, drain off the soaking water, add fresh water, and bring to a boil then simmer until beans are tender. Use the directions on the package as a time guide.
- Don't add salt to the cooking water—it slows down water absorption so cooking takes longer.
- Don't cook beans in the water they have soaked in. Substances that contribute to flatulence are leached from the beans into the soaking and cooking waters.

Canned legumes: most legumes are available canned, making cooking with beans quick and easy. One 14-ounce can of beans substitutes for ¾ cup of dried beans.

4. Include nuts regularly in your diet

Nuts are a food that most people enjoy but few people eat regularly, particularly if they are watching their weight. The good news is that a number of large studies have now shown a relationship between regular nut consumption and a reduced risk of both heart disease and type 2 diabetes. Eaten in small amounts nuts have also been shown to assist with weight control as they are satisfying and therefore stop you snacking on other foods.

Nuts are a healthy choice because they contain:

- very little saturated fat (the fats are predominantly mono- or polyunsaturated)
- dietary fiber

- vitamin E, an antioxidant believed to help prevent heart disease
- folate, copper, and magnesium, nutrients thought to protect against heart disease

Walnuts and pecans also contain some omega-3 fats, while flaxseeds are very rich in omega-3s, lignans, and plant estrogens. When freshly ground, flaxseeds have a subtle nutty flavor and make a great addition to breads, muffins, biscuits, and cereals. (Flaxseed oil is also available for use in things like salad dressings.)

Remember to choose the unsalted variety—salted nuts are usually roasted in saturated fat. And stick to a handful a day if you are watching your weight.

Some easy ways to eat more nuts include:

Breakfast

- Sprinkle a mixture of nuts and seeds over your cereal.
- Use a spread such as peanut, almond, or cashew butter on your toast in place of butter or margarine.

Lunch

- Add a handful of walnuts or pine nuts to your salad.
- Tahini (sesame seed paste) can be used as a spread on sandwiches or in salads in place of mayonnaise.

Dinner

- Add nuts and seeds to your favorite meals—try peanuts or sesame seeds in a stir-fry, cashews with a curry, or crushed macadamias with fish or chicken.
- Pesto (ground pine nuts, basil, garlic, and olive oil) makes a good pasta sauce or accompaniment to meat or fish.
- Tahini can be used as an alternative to sour cream on potatoes or drizzled over roasted vegetables.

Snacks and desserts

- Enjoy nuts as a snack. Although high in fat, nuts make a healthy substitute for less nutritious high-fat snacks such as potato chips, chocolate, and cookies. Just be careful not to eat too many—limit to one handful (about 30 grams) each day!
- Whole-grain crackers or toast with nut spread make a satisfying snack.
- Nuts and seeds can be added to baked goods—try walnuts, hazelnuts, and almond meal in cakes and muffins; and sunflower seeds, pumpkin seeds, sesame seeds, and linseeds in bread.

5. Eat more fish and seafood

Fish, particularly oily fish, are the best source of long chain omega-3 fatty acids, fats that offer valuable health benefits. These types of fats can help to reduce blood clotting and inflammatory reactions, and studies have shown that regular fish consumption is linked to a reduced risk of coronary heart disease. In fact, just one serving of fish a week may reduce the risk of a fatal heart attack by 40 percent. Our bodies only make small amounts of these fatty acids and so we rely on dietary sources, especially fish and seafood, for them. You should try to eat fish at least twice a week.

Fresh fish that contain the highest amounts of omega-3 fats include:

- swordfish
- salmon
- gemfish
- silver perch

Canned fish can also provide omega-3 fats, good sources being:

- salmon
- sardines

A Word about Fish and Mercury

Due to the risk of high levels of mercury in certain species of fish, the U.S. Food and Drug Administration (FDA) has advised that pregnant women, nursing mothers, women planning pregnancy, and young children should avoid consuming certain species but can continue to consume a variety of fish as a part of a healthy diet. Shark, swordfish, king mackerel, and tilefish should not be consumed because these long-lived, larger fish contain the highest levels of mercury. Pregnant women should select a variety of other kinds of fish—shellfish, canned fish such as light tuna, smaller ocean fish, or farm-raised fish. The FDA recommends two three-ounce servings per week, but you can safely eat up to twelve ounces of cooked fish per week.

Shopping for fish can be a bit of a minefield. For up-to-date facts and information on sustainable fish, visit www.montereybayaquarium.org/cr/seafoodwatch.aspx. You can download a printable pocket guide as well.

Try to choose varieties canned in spring water where possible. If you choose fish canned in oil, go for those in olive or canola oil.

You could easily include fish in your diet at least twice a week by having one main meal of fresh fish and a serving of canned salmon or sardines for lunch or breakfast at least once a week.

Just remember not to cook your fish in solid (saturated) fat. That means avoiding eating fried fish from fast-food restaurants, even if they say cooked in "vegetable oil." If you eat precooked breaded (crumbed) frozen-fish products choose low-fat varieties or those that have been cooked in canola oil. You can now get frozen fish products without the crumbs (e.g., Gorton's Grilled Fillets) and these would make an even better choice.

To increase your intake of fish, try the following ideas:

Breakfast

- Sardines on toast will fill you up in the morning and give you a good dose of omega-3s.
- Try an omelet with smoked salmon.

Lunch

- Add tuna or salmon to a sandwich or salad.
- For something different, try baked salmon or tuna fish cakes on a roll with lettuce and avocado.
- Grilled fish with salad makes a healthy lunch choice if eating out.

Dinner

- Homemade fish and chips is a quick and easy meal to prepare—wrap fish in foil with lemon juice and herbs and bake in the oven along with sweet potato chips (slice and brush with olive oil—bake on tray in oven). Serve with salad or steamed vegetables.
- Try adding tuna or salmon to pasta with a tomato sauce and some vegetables.
- Barbecue fish makes a healthy alternative to sausages and fatty meats.

If you don't eat fish or seafood, you can also get some omega-3 fatty acids from plant foods. Good sources include flaxseed, canola, walnut, and soybean oils. There are also small amounts in walnuts, linseeds, pecans, soybeans, baked beans, wheat germ, and green leafy vegetables.

6. Eat lean meats and low-fat dairy foods

Scientists have known for years that a diet high in saturated fat raises cholesterol levels and increases heart disease risk. More recently, research has also implicated these fats in both insulin resistance and obesity—we burn saturated fat poorly compared to other fats, so it tends to be stored as body fat more readily. In contrast, our bodies are more likely to use omega-3 polyunsaturated fatty acids (PUFAs) and monounsaturated fatty acids (MUFAs) for energy rather than storage.

Reducing your intake of saturated fat doesn't mean that you need to avoid red meat and dairy products. They are good sources of protein, iron, and calcium, so as long as you choose lean cuts of meat and low-fat dairy products you can still include these foods in moderation as part of a healthy diet.

If you enjoy meat, we suggest eating lean red meat two or three times a week, and accompanying it with salad and vegetables. Trim all visible fat from meat and remove the skin (and the fat just below it) from chicken. Game meats such as rabbit and venison are not only lean but are also good sources of omega-3 fatty acids, as are organ meats such as liver and kidney. If you choose not to eat red meat or are trying to reduce your intake, legumes and tofu are a good alternative as they can provide the protein, iron, and zinc that's also found in red meat.

Replacing full fat dairy foods with reduced-fat, low-fat, or fat-free varieties will also help you reduce your saturated fat intake. Dairy products including milk, yogurt, and cheese are among the richest sources of calcium in our diet. They also provide protein, and a number of important vitamins and minerals including vitamin B_{12}, phosphorous, magnesium, and zinc.

Alternatively you could choose calcium-fortified soy products such as soy milk and soy yogurt. Soy products contain mostly polyunsaturated fat and the protein in soy products can help to lower cholesterol levels. Soy products are also a source of omega-3 fatty acids and phytoestrogens. Much of the saturated fat we consume these days comes from pre-prepared packaged and fast-food meals; in fact, most fast-food restaurants cook with saturated fat (from either animal or vegetable sources).

Phytoestrogens: Protection from Plants

Phytoestrogens are natural plant chemicals found in foods such as fruit, vegetables, nuts, and soy foods. Research shows that people who consume high levels of phytoestrogens enjoy better health and live longer. Phytoestrogens can help to reduce the symptoms of menopause and can lower cholesterol levels and protect against cancer. You can increase your intake of phytoestrogens by eating legumes, tofu, and nuts regularly, switching from dairy to soy milk and eating breads and cereals containing soy and linseed.

Until these restaurants make an effort to reduce the saturated fat content of their products, it's best to eat as little fried fast food as possible.

We used to think that eating high cholesterol foods such as eggs, shrimp, and other shellfish would raise our blood cholesterol levels. We now know that our liver compensates for the increased cholesterol intake by reducing cholesterol production, although a small percentage of people have an inherited condition called familial hypercholesterolemia, which impairs this self-regulation. This means that most people could eat an egg a day, for example, without harming their heart.

To enhance your intake of omega-3 fats we suggest that you eat omega-3 enriched eggs (if you can find them), which have about six times more ALA and DHA than regular eggs. These enriched eggs are produced by feeding the hens a diet that is naturally rich in omega-3s (including canola and linseeds).

You can include lean meats and low-fat dairy products in your diet in the following ways:

Breakfast

- Try poached or scrambled eggs on toast or an omelet.
- Fruit smoothies make a great breakfast when you are on the go. If you don't have time to make your own, try Odwalla Real Fruit Smoothies.
- Low-fat yogurt is a tasty accompaniment to muesli.

Lunch

- Sandwiches or rolls can be filled with chicken and avocado, lean roast beef and mustard, turkey and cranberry, sliced lamb with hummus, egg and lettuce, or lean ham and salad.
- If you prefer toasted sandwiches try chicken and avocado, ham, cheese and tomato, or ricotta, sun-dried tomato, and arugula. Dress up your salad with lean roast meat, sliced chicken breast, a boiled egg, or some cubes of low-fat feta cheese.

Why Do I Never See a GI Value for Meat or Cheese?

The foods we eat contain three main nutrients—protein, carbohydrate, and fat. Some foods, such as meat, are high in protein, while bread is high in carbohydrate and butter is high in fat. It is necessary for us to consume a variety of foods (in varying proportions) to provide all three nutrients, but the GI applies only to foods containing carbohydrate. It is impossible for us to measure a GI value for foods that contain negligible carbohydrate. These foods include meat, fish, chicken, eggs, cheese, nuts, oils, cream, butter, and most vegetables. There are other nutritional aspects that you could consider in choosing these foods, for example the amount and type of fats they contain.

- Frittata made with eggs, low-fat milk, chopped vegetables, lean ham, fresh herbs, and low-fat cheese makes a tasty weekend lunch or brunch served with salad.
- Soups are a great winter warmer. Try chicken and sweet corn, beef and vegetable, or lamb shank and barley.
- For a variation on your usual sandwich, try a pita bread filled with hummus, tabbouli, and sliced chicken breast or roast lamb.

Dinner

- Go for lean meats—marinated and grilled, or pan-fried with a little olive or canola oil.
- Beef and chicken can be sliced into strips and stir-fried with vegetables.
- For the barbecue choose lean steak, marinated chicken breast, or kebabs.
- Use lean meats in curries and casseroles and if you have time cook the day before, refrigerate, and skim fat from top the next day before reheating to serve.
- Low-fat yogurt and ricotta mixed with chives makes a low-fat alternative to sour cream on vegetables or Mexican food.

Snacks and desserts

- Fruit smoothies or low-fat milkshakes make a satisfying calcium-packed snack.
- Yogurt is always a quick and easy option.
- Try a glass of chocolate Nesquik or a low-fat hot chocolate to satisfy those chocolate cravings.
- Low-fat flavored milk or soy milks make a good snack on the run.
- Ricotta can be used as topping for crackers or spread on fruit loaf.
- Add a spoonful of low-fat pudding, frozen yogurt, or ice-cream to fruit for dessert.
- Low-fat ricotta can also be used in cheesecakes or as a topping for fresh fruit.

7. Use high omega-3 and monounsaturated oils such as olive, peanut, and canola oils

It's not necessary, or beneficial, to cut all fats out of your diet. In fact, some fat is essential for our health to provide essential fatty acids and for carrying fat-soluble vitamins and antioxidants. This means that it's fine to use small amounts of oil in cooking and salad dressings, but it's important to choose the right one. If you don't use oil you could also get these "good" fats from eating nuts, seeds, avocado, olives, and fish.

When choosing oil, you want to choose types that are high in monounsaturated and omega-3 fats. These include:

Olive oil is high in monounsaturated fats and low in saturates with a minimal polyunsaturated fat content, which is an advantage as it allows our bodies to make greater use of the omega-3 fats we obtain from other dietary sources, without any competition from excessive polyunsaturated omega-6 fats. Olive oil is also rich in antioxidants that have many health benefits. Olive oil can be used in cooking and is the best choice for salad dressings. Olive oil margarines are also available.

Types of Fats and Their Sources

There is less evidence to support reducing the amount of fat we eat than there is to recommend changing the type. Although foods contain a mixture of fatty acids, one type of fatty acid tends to predominate, allowing us to categorize foods according to their main fatty acid component. It is best to choose monounsaturated and polyunsaturated fats in place of saturated.

An asterisk next to a food in the following list means the food is a good source of omega-3 fatty acids.

Polyunsaturated products

Oils
Safflower, sunflower, grapeseed, soybean*, corn, flaxseed*, cottonseed, walnut*, sesame, evening primrose oils

Spreads
Polyunsaturated margarines, tahini (sesame seed paste)

Nuts and seeds
Walnuts*, sunflower seeds, pumpkin seeds, sesame seeds

Other plant sources
Soybeans, soy milk, wheat germ, whole grains

Animal sources
Oily fish*

Monounsaturated products

Oils
Olive, canola*, peanut, rapeseed oil, macadamia, and mustard seed oils

Spreads
Olive oil margarines, canola margarine*, peanut butter

Nuts and seeds
Cashews, macadamias, almonds, hazelnuts, pecans, pistachio, peanuts

Other plant sources
Avocado, olives

Animal sources
Very lean red meat, lean chicken, lean pork, egg yolks
Saturated products

Saturated Products

Oils/Fats
Palm and palm kernel oil, coconut oil, drippings, lard, ghee, solid frying oils, cooking margarines, and shortening

Spreads
Butter, cream cheese

Dairy foods
Full-fat dairy products: cheese, cream, sour cream, yogurt, whole milk, ice cream

Animal sources
Fat on beef, lamb, skin on chicken, sausage, salami, most luncheon meats

Peanut oil is a mild-tasting oil that oxidizes slowly and can withstand high cooking temperatures. About 50 percent of the fat in peanut oil is monounsaturated and another 30 percent is polyunsaturated. This heart-healthy fat is good for Asian cooking such as stir-fries.

Canola oil, besides being high in monounsaturated fat, canola contains significant amounts of omega-3 fats. Canola oil is a multipurpose cooking oil and can also be used for baking cakes and muffins. Margarine made from canola oil is also available.

Flaxseed oil (also known as linseed) is the richest plant source of omega-3s and contains very little omega-6 fats. But flaxseed oil is highly prone to oxidation (meaning the fats it contains turn rancid easily) so it shouldn't be heated and needs to be stored carefully. It is best used in a salad dressing. Alternatively, linseeds can be freshly ground and sprinkled on cereal or added to cakes and muffins.

Rapeseed oil, commonly marketed under the name canola oil, is another highly monounsaturated oil, making it an ideal alternative to the saturated fats that manufacturers normally use for frying. It is now being used by some food manufacturers to produce healthier fast-food choices. Like canola oil, it contains significant amounts of omega-3 fats.

Cold-pressed? Virgin? Extra virgin? Light? Extra light?

Cold-pressed oils are those that have undergone minimal processing—this means that the oil is extracted from the seed, nut, or fruit by mechanical pressing only, without heat or solvents. Cold-pressed oils have a stronger flavor and color than their regular counterparts, and they're also much richer in vitamin E (a natural preservative present in oils) and other antioxidants, giving them important health benefits. For example, extra-virgin olive oil—the best quality oil made from the first cold-pressing of the olives—contains 30 to 40 different antioxidants. It is dark-colored and strong in flavor.

Light and extra-light oils are light in color and flavor. The terms "light" and "extra light" don't mean, however, that the oil is lower in fat than any other oil—all oils are 100 percent fat.

I was referred to the doctor for severe hypothyroidism. Although within a few weeks a thyroid hormone brought my thyroid tests to normal, I did not lose the weight I had put on and my periods remained really unpredictable. My doctor ran serum prolactin, FSH, and LH tests. The prolactin was abnormal, twice the upper limit of the normal range, but an MRI of the pituitary gland to diagnose (or exclude) a pituitary growth was inconclusive. Over the next few months the prolactin peaked again, and this time my doctor suspected that it may be linked to PCOS, which an internal ultrasound scan confirmed. He prescribed metformin and at the same time I saw a dietitian who reviewed my diet and put me on a healthy low-GI eating program. I lost 14 pounds in three weeks and have to say that I shouted from the rooftops that I have never eaten as much, nor felt as well. . . . All the energy that I thought I had lost has come back!
Juliet, 34

Should I Avoid All High-GI Foods?

I am confused. Chocolate has a low GI and watermelon is high—does this mean I should choose chocolate over watermelon as a snack?

The GI of a food does not make it good or bad for us. High-GI foods like potato and bread still make a valuable nutritional contribution to our diet. And low-GI foods like pastry or chocolate that are high in saturated fat are no better for us because of their low GI. The nutritional benefits of different foods are many and varied, and it is advisable for you to base your food choices on the overall nutritional content of a food, particularly considering the saturated fat, salt, fiber, and GI values.

The flavor on fluids

An adequate fluid intake is essential for good health, but most people don't drink enough. Most adults need about 2 liters of fluid each day (about 8 glasses) to replace the fluid that is lost from the body. More is needed in hot weather, during exercise, and if you work in air-conditioning. An adequate fluid intake is important for kidney function, temperature regulation, and for preventing constipation.

Water is the best fluid to quench your thirst and is also the best choice if you are watching your weight and insulin levels. Soft drinks, energy drinks, and cordials contain large amounts of added sugar and it is best to avoid these where possible. Most fruit juices have a relatively low GI and can be consumed in moderation, but remember that they still contain a lot of carbohydrate from the natural fruit sugars.

It would be better to eat the whole fruit (which still contains the fiber) rather than drinking the juice.

If you struggle to drink plain water you could try mineral or soda water with a slice of lemon or lime and a few fresh mint leaves. Or try diluting fruit juice with water, soda water, or mineral water. Tea is also fine—green tea, in particular, has been shown to be high in antioxidants. If you like hot drinks, there are also a wide variety of herbal teas available, but if you are pregnant you need to be careful as some types are not suitable during pregnancy.

Coffee and alcohol have a diuretic effect so should not be counted as part of your 8 glasses. Both are best consumed in moderation. Alcohol is also high in calories so should be limited when watching your weight. The recommendation for women is to limit alcoholic drinks to one or fewer drinks per day.

Milk and soy milk are low GI but it is best to choose low-fat varieties, particularly when weight loss is a goal. If you don't like the taste of milk or soy milk on their own, you could add a teaspoon of chocolate Nesquik or drinking chocolate for flavor, or make a fruit smoothie for a satisfying snack or breakfast on the run.

A quick guide to healthy low-GI eating

If you are looking for ways to improve your diet, there are two important things to remember.

1. Identify the sources of carbohydrates in your diet and reduce high-GI foods. Don't go to extremes; there is still room for your favorite high-GI foods.

   Some of the most common changes women tell us they have made to achieve a low-GI diet are:

   - swapping white and wheat flour breads for the whole-grain varieties
   - choosing low-GI breakfast cereals like oats
   - eating more fruit and yogurt in place of other snack foods
   - adding more legumes to meals
   - choosing more sweet potato, corn, and legumes in place of white potato

2. Identify the sources of fat in your diet and look at ways you can reduce saturated fat. Choose monounsaturated and polyunsaturated fats, such as olive oil and sunflower oil, instead of saturated fats like butter and shortening. The body needs some fat, and there's room for your favorite fatty foods on occasion—just remember to watch your portions.

Substituting High-GI Foods
with Low-GI Alternatives

High-GI food	Low-GI alternative
Bread—white or wheat flour	Bread containing lots of grains such as Shiloh Farms Sprouted 7-grain, French Meadow Bakery 100% rye and sunflower seed, or Arnold stone-ground 100% whole wheat
Processed breakfast cereals	Unrefined cereals such as rolled oats or muesli or a low-GI processed cereal like All-Bran or Bran Buds.
Plain biscuits or crackers	Biscuits made with dried fruit, oats, and whole grains, e.g., Quaker chewy granola bars, Kudos whole-grain bars, and Ryvita fruit crispbread
Cakes and Muffins	Make them with fruit, oats, and whole grains
Potato	Substitute with baby new potatoes, sweet potato, sweet corn
Rice	Try longer grain varieties such as basmati, Uncle Ben's converted, long-grain rice, and Uncle Ben's long-grain and wild rice blend, or try pearled barley or noodles instead

A few simple changes you could make to reduce your intake of saturated fat are:

- use avocado, hummus, or nut spreads in place of butter
- choose lean meats and eat more fish and legumes in place of red meat
- choose low-fat dairy products or try a calcium-fortified soy product instead
- snack on fruit, yogurt, dried fruit, nuts, and hummus with vegetables in place of higher fat snack foods like potato chips, cakes, and biscuits

Putting it all together—a typical day the low-GI way

We hope that having read this far you now have a good idea of how to build low-GI foods into your diet. But just in case you're still not sure, it should look something like this:

Breakfast

Breakfast is the most important meal of the day—it gets your metabolism going and prevents you getting hungry and snacking on high-fat foods later in the morning. Research has shown that people who eat breakfast regularly find it easier to lose weight and have better energy levels and concentration throughout the day. If you are always in a rush in the morning, it's well worth making the time for breakfast— 5 or 10 minutes is all it takes.

Step 1: Choose high-fiber cereal based on oats and barley or heavy whole-grain breads such as such as Shiloh Farms Sprouted 7-grain, French Meadow Bakery 100 percent rye and sunflower seed, or Arnold stone-ground 100 percent whole wheat.

Step 2: Add some protein to keep you satisfied for longer. Good choices include low-fat milk or yogurt, canned fish, baked beans, eggs, ricotta or cottage cheese, and nuts or nut spreads.

Step 3: Toss in some fruit or vegetables for a healthy dose of fiber, vitamins, and antioxidants. Try berries with muesli and yogurt, old-fashioned oatmeal with stewed apple, grilled tomatoes and mushrooms with eggs, or asparagus on toast.

Try these suggestions for a tasty, satisfying breakfast:

- Bircher muesli with yogurt and berries
- Whole-grain toast with natural almond spread
- Oatmeal with soy milk and stewed apple
- Sardines and tomato on whole-grain toast
- A bowl of low-GI cereal (try unrefined cereals such as rolled oats or muesli or a low-GI processed cereal like All-Bran or Bran Buds) with low-fat milk or soy milk
- Fruit salad with yogurt and a sprinkle of natural muesli
- Toasted rye sourdough with ricotta and tomato
- Soy milk berry smoothie
- Hummus on 9-grain English muffins
- Homemade apple, walnut, and oat bran muffin

Lunch

Taking a break for a satisfying lunchtime meal is important for maintaining energy levels and concentration and preventing hunger and excessive snacking during the afternoon and early evening. Whether you are eating at home, taking lunch with you, or buying a meal out, there are plenty of healthy choices available.

Step 1: Pick your low GI carbs. Try a whole-grain bread or roll, Ryvita crispbreads, pasta or noodles, low-GI rice, quinoa, legumes, or cracked wheat.

Step 2: Add a good serving of vegetables or salad.

Step 3: Finish with a small amount of lean protein. Good choices include canned fish, eggs, lean chicken or turkey, leftover cold meat from dinner, marinated tofu, ricotta or cottage cheese, and legumes. Avoid processed and smoked meats and fish, which are high in salt and have been linked with an increased risk of type 2 diabetes and cancer.

The options are endless, but here are a few ideas to get you started:

- Whole-grain sandwich with salmon and salad
- Garden salad with chicken, avocado, and croutons made from whole-grain bread cut into cubes and baked in the oven. Dress with a mixture of olive oil, vinegar, and lemon juice
- Vietnamese rice paper rolls filled with vegetables and tofu or prawns
- Vegetable frittata made with sweet potato, capsicum, peas, and corn
- Bowl of minestrone or lentil and vegetable soup (preferably homemade)
- Asparagus and capsicum bread quiches. Use whole-grain bread rolled out and pressed into muffin tins in place of pastry
- Toasted sourdough with ricotta and roasted vegetables (try red pepper, eggplant, zucchini, and pumpkin)

- Low-GI multigrain wrap with falafel, hummus, and tabbouli
- Ryvita crispbread with tuna, tomato, and cucumber
- Tuna pasta salad—combine cold pasta spirals and canned tuna in spring water, snow peas, and cherry tomatoes and make a dressing from natural yogurt, lemon juice, and fresh herbs
- Mini-muffin pizzas using 9-grain multi-grain English muffins, topped with tomato, red and green pepper, mushrooms, and a sprinkle of grated mozzarella
- Roasted vegetable salad (try red or green peppers, zucchini, pumpkin or sweet potato, eggplant brushed with olive oil and baked in the oven) with chickpeas, baby spinach leaves, and a dash of balsamic vinegar

Dinner

When you are tired after a long day, it can be hard to get motivated to cook. Fortunately, putting a meal together at the end of the day doesn't have to take a lot of time and effort, as you will see with our recipes. The key is to have your kitchen well stocked with the right foods—use our shopping list to make sure you have everything you need.

Step 1: Fill half of your plate with a variety of different non-starchy vegetables or salads. Aim to make your plate as colorful as possible.

Step 2: Fill another quarter of your plate with some low-fat protein—fish, seafood, lean meat, skinless poultry, eggs, tofu, or legumes.

Step 3: Fill the remaining quarter of your plate with low-GI carbs—pasta, noodles, basmati rice, barley, quinoa, cracked wheat, corn, orange sweet potato, or legumes.

Step 4: For flavor, use fresh or dried herbs and spices, garlic, ginger, chili, lemon and lime juice, vinegar, olive oil, no-added-salt canned crushed tomatoes or tomato paste. Avoid most pre-prepared sauces (particularly stir-through and simmer sauces in which you add the whole jar), as these are usually high in fat, sugar, or salt.

Here are just a few examples:

- Small grilled lean steak with cob of corn and garden salad
- Baked salmon fillet with homemade oven fries (using new potatoes, sliced and brushed with olive oil) and steamed carrot, broccoli, and beans
- Quinoa with roasted vegetables (such as red pepper, eggplant, zucchini, and pumpkin) and chickpeas
- Lean meat rissoles with potato and cannellini bean mash, beans, peas, and carrots
- Tofu and vegetable stir-fry with Hokkien noodles
- Lean lamb kebabs with tabbouli, hummus, and salad
- Barley risotto with mushrooms, capsicum, spinach, peas, and sliced chicken breast
- Spinach and ricotta cannelloni with salad
- Chicken and lentil curry with basmati rice and steamed greens
- Corn tortillas filled with a mixture of lean mince and kidney beans (with onion, garlic, chili, and canned crushed tomatoes) and chopped tomato, lettuce, cucumber, and mashed avocado

Snacks

There is nothing wrong with eating between meals if you are hungry. In fact, eating three small meals and two to three snacks rather than three big meals can help to keep blood glucose and insulin levels more stable over the day. But most processed snack foods are high in fat, sugar, or salt and are best left on the shelf. If you are cutting energy to lose weight but also want to get all the nutrients your body needs, it is important to choose nutrient-dense snack foods and avoid "empty calories."

Good choices include:

- A serving of fresh fruit
- A small handful of raw nuts (30–40g)
- A small bowl of berries with 2 tbsp. of natural yogurt
- 2–3 Ryvita crackers with cottage cheese and tomato
- 2 tbsp. tzatziki or hummus dip (look for lower fat and salt varieties or make your own) with raw carrot and celery
- 1 slice of whole-grain fruit bread with low-fat ricotta
- A handful of roasted chickpeas
- A small container of low-fat yogurt

Eating out

Many of the women we see comment that they find eating out difficult. We recognize that it can be harder when you don't have control over your food choices, but there are many options that fit the low-GI way of eating.

Try these:

- Asian: steamed, braised, or stir-fried dishes with noodles
- Indian: Tandoori, dahl, vegetable, and legume curries with basmati rice
- Mexican: tacos, burritos, or tortillas with beans, salad, guacamole, and a sprinkle of cheese (avoid the sour cream)
- Italian: small pasta with a tomato, pesto, or seafood sauce served with a side salad
- pizza: gourmet-style thin crust with vegetarian or seafood topping
- pita bread or falafel roll with hummus and tabbouli
- plain hamburger with lots of salad on a whole-grain roll (leave the butter)
- Barbecue chicken (remove the skin) with a cob of corn and a side salad instead of chips
- Vietnamese rice paper rolls

While we suggest trying to include at least one low-GI food with each meal, this may not always be possible when eating out. One option is to combine a high-GI food with a low-GI food to give a moderate effect—for example, rice with legumes or potato with corn. If this is not possible, just have a small serving of the higher-GI food and fill up with plenty of vegetables and salads. And, remember, if it is only once in a while it really won't matter. If you eat out a few times each week, you will need to be more careful.

Your healthy low-GI shopping list

To make low-GI choices easy choices, you need to stock your pantry with the right foods. Here are some ideas of what to include on your shopping list:

Breads

Rudolph's Specialty Bakeries linseed and rye
Shiloh Farms sprouted 7-grain
French Meadow Bakery 100% rye and sunflower seed
Alvarado Street Bakery 100% sprouted sourdough, barley, or
    raisin bread
Arnold stone-ground 100% whole wheat
Pepperidge Farm Sprouted Wheat
Healthy Choice Hearty 7-grain
Vermont Bread Company 100% whole wheat

Breakfast cereals

Rolled oats (whole or old-fashioned, not instant)
All-Bran, All-Bran Fruit & Oats (Kellogg's)
Bran Buds, Bran Buds with psyllium (Kellogg's)
Natural muesli
Special K (Kellogg's)
    Zoe Foods flax and soy cereal with almonds and oats

Rice, pasta, and grains

Basmati, Uncle Ben's converted, long-grain rice, and Uncle Ben's
    long-grain and wild rice blend
Pasta—fresh or dried
Noodles
Pearl barley
Cracked wheat
Quinoa

Legumes

Dried legumes, e.g., lentils, split peas, chickpeas, kidney beans, cannellini beans

Canned legumes, e.g., kidney beans; three- or four-bean mix

Baked beans

Pinto beans, black beans

Vegetables

All fresh, frozen, and canned vegetables

All salad vegetables

Canned tomatoes

Sweet potato, corn, yam, baby new potato

Fruits

All fruits are suitable, but the lowest GI varieties include:

Apples

Cherries

Grapefruit

Grapes

Kiwi fruit

Oranges

Pears

Plums

Peaches

Dried fruit including apricots, raisins, apples, prunes, and pears

Canned fruits in natural juice

Fruit snack packs

Fruit juices (limited to 1–2 glasses per day)

Meats

Lean cuts such as trim beef, lamb and veal, new-fashion pork

Skinless chicken or turkey

Low-fat, lean, ground meats

Fish and seafood

All fresh fish

Canned fish including salmon, sardines, tuna, mackerel, and herring

Smoked fish such as smoked cod and smoked salmon

Frozen fish products without crumbs (e.g., Gorton's Grilled Fillets) or made with poly- or monounsaturated oils (check the label)

Most seafood except battered or crumbed

Dairy foods or nondairy alternatives

Reduced-fat or skim milk

Calcium-fortified soy milk

Low-fat or nonfat yogurts

Soy yogurts

UHT or powdered skim milk for cooking

Canned evaporated skim milk

Low-fat ice cream or soy ice cream

Cottage cheese, low-fat ricotta cheese

Low-fat flavored milks or soy milks

Low-fat cheese: block, slices, or grated for cooking

Spreads

If you use a spread, choose one labeled "polyunsaturated" or "monounsaturated," and preferably one that is salt reduced. Alternatively try using avocado, hummus, tahini (sesame seed spread), or nut butters—these contain good types of fats as well as providing a variety of vitamins and minerals.

Flavors, sauces, oils, and dressings

Fresh and dried herbs

Spices

Cold-pressed olive oil, canola, peanut oil, or flaxseed oil

Vinegar: white wine, red wine, and balsamic

Curry powders and pastes

Bottled tomato pasta sauces and tomato paste

Sauces including soy, oyster, sweet chili, hoisin, and fish

Bottled minced ginger, garlic, and chili
Lemon and lime juice
Black pepper
Mustard
Sun-dried tomatoes, olives, artichoke hearts

PCOS Kickstart Diet

In general, we don't find that set menu plans work for most people, as they are hard to follow, unless of course you have had an individualized menu plan developed specifically for you. However, we also know that some people like to have a "diet" to follow, particularly when they are getting started. So we have put together our "Kickstart" menus to help fast-track your success. Try this for the first few weeks, but then we hope you will use our meal planning guidelines to add more variety and develop your own healthy eating plan for life.

The menus follow our seven dietary guidelines and emphasize fruits, vegetables, legumes, whole-grain and low-GI breads and cereals, lean meats and seafood, low-fat dairy products, and healthy oils. They also incorporate the recipes we have included in this book, which are marked with an asterisk.

We have not included serving sizes, as everyone has different energy needs and appetites. Start by focusing on making healthier food choices rather than worrying about amounts, and if you need more specific advice, we suggest that you see a Registered Dietitian (details of how to contact an RD can be found on page 35).

Kickstart Menu

	Breakfast	Morning Snack	Lunch
MONDAY	Mixed-grain oatmeal with dried fruit compote and yogurt*	Fruit	Garden salad with sliced chicken breast and whole-grain roll
TUESDAY	Fruit smoothie with strawberries, low-fat milk and yogurt	Quaker chewy granola bar	Pita bread with hummus, salad, and falafel
WEDNESDAY	Whole-grain toast with avocado and tomato	Fruit	Thick vegetable soup
THURSDAY	Natural toasted muesli* with yogurt	Handful of roasted chickpeas	Whole-grain sandwich with chicken, avocado, and salad
FRIDAY	All-Bran with sliced banana and low-fat milk	Fruit	Tuna and bean salad with garlic pita toasts*
SATURDAY	Ricotta-blueberry hotcakes*	Fruit	Chicken and mango rice paper rolls*
SUNDAY	Whole-grain toast with poached egg and steamed spinach	Fruit	Lamb burgers with sweet potato chips and spinach salad

	Afternoon Snack	Dinner
MONDAY	Handful of raw nuts	Tomato fettucine with salmon
TUESDAY	Low-fat yogurt	Balsamic lamb* with sweet potato mash, steamed beans
WEDNESDAY	Wasa sourdough rye crispbread with ricotta and tomato	Mediterranean chicken*
THURSDAY	Berries and low-fat yogurt	Grilled fish and white bean salsa with salad*
FRIDAY	9-grain English muffin with ricotta and tomato	Grilled beef with Thai noodle salad*
SATURDAY	Hummus with baked pita bread, carrot, and celery	Pork with creamy mustard sauce*
SUNDAY	Low-fat fruit smoothie	Tofu and vegetable noodles*

Kickstart Vegetarian Menu

	Breakfast	*Morning Snack*	*Lunch*
MONDAY	Natural toasted muesli with yogurt*	Fruit	Thai noodle salad with tofu
TUESDAY	Fruit smoothie with strawberries and low-fat soy milk and yogurt	Quaker chewy granola bar	Pita bread with hummus, salad, and falafel
WEDNESDAY	Whole-grain toast with avocado and tomato	Fruit	Thick vegetable soup*
THURSDAY	Natural toasted muesli with yogurt*	Handful of roasted chickpeas	Whole-grain roll with lentil burger, avocado, and salad
FRIDAY	Mixed-grain oatmeal with dried fruit compote and yogurt*	Fruit	Chickpea and beetroot salad* with sprouted wheat bread
SATURDAY	Scrambled tofu with grilled tomato and whole-grain toast	Fruit	Carrot, avocado, and snow pea rice paper rolls*
SUNDAY	Sweet corn and mushroom omelette*	Fruit	Bean and corn burritos*

For a vegan diet:

- Replace milk and yogurt with soy milk and soy yogurt (preferably fortified with calcium and vitamin B12)
- Replace ricotta in cannelloni with silken tofu

	Afternoon Snack	*Dinner*
MONDAY	Handful of raw nuts	Lentil and ricotta cannelloni with baby spinach
TUESDAY	Low-fat yogurt	Fennel, leek and bean barley pilaf*
WEDNESDAY	Wasa sourdough rye crispbread with ricotta and tomato	3-bean chili with spicy tortilla crisps*
THURSDAY	Berries and low-fat yogurt	Shitake, ginger and tofu hokiien noodles*
FRIDAY	Berry soy smoothie	Stuffed vegetables*
SATURDAY	Hummus with baked pita bread, carrot, and celery	Morrocan chickpea and lentil soup*
SUNDAY	Low-fat fruit smoothie	Chargrilled vegetable and tofu salad*

For a vegan diet:
- Replace ricotta as spread with avocado, hummus, or almond butter
- Replace hard cheese with soy cheese or omit
- Replace omelette with scrambled tofu or baked beans

Kickstart Gluten-Free Menu

	Breakfast	Morning Snack	Lunch
MONDAY	Multi-grain porridge*	Fruit	Tangy tuna rice paper rolls
TUESDAY	Fruit smoothie with strawberries, low-fat milk and yogurt	Fruit	Chickpea and beetroot salad* with whole-grain gluten-free bread
WEDNESDAY	Whole-grain gluten-free toast with ricotta and tomato	Fruit	Moroccan bean and lentil soup*
THURSDAY	Gluten-free muesli* with low-fat natural yogurt	Handful of roasted chickpeas	Chicken and mango rice paper rolls
FRIDAY	Quinoa porridge with low-fat milk and banana	Fruit	Tuna and bean salad with gluten-free garlic toast
SATURDAY	Sweet corn and mushroom omelette with gluten-free whole-grain toast	Fruit	Grilled beef with Thai noodle salad*
SUNDAY	Multi-grain porridge*	Fruit	Bean and corn burritos*

Notes for GF menu:

- Choose lower GI gluten-free breads and cereals where available
- Choose gluten-free stock for soups

	Afternoon Snack	Dinner
MONDAY	Handful of raw nuts	Shitake ginger and tofu soba noodles*
TUESDAY	Low-fat yogurt	Balsamic lamb* with sweet potato mash, steamed beans and baby squash
WEDNESDAY	Whole-grain gluten-free toast with ricotta and tomato	Salmon and squash patties with lima bean salad*
THURSDAY	Berries and low-fat yogurt	Grilled fish and white bean salsa with salad*
FRIDAY	Handful of dried fruit and nuts	Lamb cutlets with pea pilaf*
SATURDAY	Hummus with carrot and celery	Pork with creamy mustard sauce*
SUNDAY	Low-fat fruit smoothie	Grilled lemon chicked skewers* with pistachio and quinoa tabbouli*

Notes for GF menu:

- Use gluten-free buckwheat soba noodles in place of Hokkien noodles (Monday dinner)
- Use gluten-free flatbreads in place of pita bread for garlic toasts (lunch Friday)

7
Recipes

Breakfasts

MIXED-GRAIN OATMEAL WITH DRIED FRUIT COMPOTE AND YOGURT

Per serving: Calories 258 ■ Protein 9 g ■ Fat 2.5 g (saturated fat 0.5 g)
Carbohydrate 50 g

GI LOW

Serves 4 ■ Preparation time: 10 minutes ■ Cooking time: 15 minutes

⅔ cup dried apples
⅓ cup dried apricots
¼ cup pitted prunes
4 cups water
1 cinnamon stick
¾ cup rolled oats
¾ cup rolled barley
6½ oz. Stonyfield Farm low-fat vanilla yogurt, to serve

1. Combine the apples, apricots, prunes, 1 cup of water, and the cinnamon stick in a medium-sized saucepan. Bring to a boil, then reduce the heat, partially cover and simmer for 10–15 minutes, or until the fruit is soft. Discard the cinnamon stick and cool slightly.
2. Meanwhile, place the oats and barley in another medium-sized saucepan and add 3 cups of water. Bring to a boil, then reduce the heat and simmer for 3–5 minutes, stirring frequently, until creamy.
3. Spoon the oatmeal into serving bowls, top with the fruit compote and drizzle with some of the fruit cooking liquid. Add a dollop of yogurt and serve immediately.

Note: The compote can be made up to three days in advance. Refrigerate until required, then reheat, or serve cold.

MULTI-GRAIN PORRIDGE WITH APPLE

There's nothing better on a cold morning than a warm breakfast. Enjoy this combination of grains and nuts as is or, if you wish, add a tablespoon or two of raisins for extra texture. We like using cloudy apple juice because research shows it has almost four times more antioxidants than clear juice. And it's naturally sweet, so you don't need to top the porridge with extra sugar or honey.

Per Serving: Calories 265 ■ Protein 8 g ■ Fiber 3.5 g
Fat 7 g (including 1.5 g saturated fat) ■ Carbohydrate 42 g

GI LOW

Serves 4 ■ Preparation time: 5 minutes ■ Cooking time: 5 minutes

⅓ cup quinoa flakes
⅓ cup brown rice flakes
½ teaspoon ground cinnamon
1½ tablespoons rice bran
2½ cups cloudy apple juice
2 teaspoons psyllium husks
¼ cup finely chopped mixed nuts (almonds, cashews, Brazil nuts, macadamias, hazelnuts, walnuts)

To Serve
1 cup low-fat milk or gluten-free soy milk
⅓ cup low-fat plain or flavored yogurt (optional)

1. Place the quinoa flakes, rice flakes, cinnamon, rice bran, and juice in a saucepan, and bring to a boil over medium heat. Reduce the heat to low and simmer gently for 2–3 minutes, stirring occasionally, or until the liquid is absorbed and you have a creamy porridge.

2. Remove from heat and stir in the psyllium husks and finely chopped nuts. Spoon the porridge into breakfast bowls and serve with milk and a tablespoon of yogurt.

NATURAL TOASTED MUESLI

While this muesli is relatively high in fat, most of it comes from the "healthy" fats in the nuts and seeds.

Per serving: Calories 304 ■ Protein 9 g ■ Fat 12 g (saturated fat 1 g)
Carbohydrate 41 g

GI LOW

Serves 12 ■ Preparation time: 15 minutes ■ Cooking time: 30 minutes
(plus 30 minutes cooling time)

2 ½ cups rolled oats
2 cups rolled rye
½ cup raw unsalted pumpkin seeds
⅓ cup sunflower seeds
¼ cup almonds, chopped
¼ cup hazelnuts, chopped
1 cup dried apricots, chopped
1 cup raisins

1. Preheat the oven to 350°F.
2. Place the oats, rye, seeds, and nuts in a large baking dish and mix until well combined.
3. Bake for 35 minutes, until lightly toasted, stirring several times during cooking.
4. Cool completely, then stir in the apricots and raisins. Serve with low-fat milk or yogurt, and fresh fruit in season. Keep the muesli in an airtight container and store in a cool, dark place for up to one month.

SOURDOUGH FRENCH TOAST WITH PEACHES

Per serving: Calories 226 ■ Protein 12 g ■ Fat 5.5 g (saturated fat 1.5 g)
Carbohydrate 31 g

GI LOW

Serves 4 ■ Preparation time: 10 minutes ■ Cooking time: 8 minutes

2 eggs
1 cup low-fat milk
1 tablespoon maple syrup
pinch nutmeg
olive oil spray
4 slices of Alvarado sprouted sourdough French bread, each about ¾-inch thick
4 fresh peaches, sliced

1. Whisk the eggs, milk, maple syrup, and nutmeg together in a shallow bowl. Lightly spray a nonstick frying pan and heat over a medium heat.

2. Dip the bread in the egg mixture and turn to coat completely. Place the bread in the heated pan and cook for 2–3 minutes on each side until golden brown. Set aside and keep warm.

3. Spray the pan lightly again, and cook the peach slices for 1–2 minutes on each side, until just softened. Serve the French toast topped with the peaches.

RICOTTA BLUEBERRY HOTCAKES

Keep cooked hotcakes warm on a plate covered with foil in a very low oven (about 250°F) while cooking the remaining batter.

Per serving: Calories 262 ■ Protein 15 g ■ Fat 8 g (saturated fat 3.5 g) Carbohydrate 32 g

GI MEDIUM

Serves 4 ■ Preparation time: 10 minutes ■ Cooking time: 7 minutes

5 oz. reduced-fat fresh ricotta
2 eggs, separated
½ cup low-fat milk
2 tablespoons granulated sugar
1 teaspoon vanilla extract
½ cup stone-ground whole wheat self-rising flour
1 cup fresh or frozen blueberries
olive oil spray
6½ oz. Stonyfield Farm low-fat French vanilla yogurt, to serve

1. Place the ricotta in a large mixing bowl and mash with a fork. Add the egg yolks, milk, sugar, and vanilla and mix with a wooden spoon to combine. Add the flour and fold in with a large metal spoon or rubber spatula until just combined. Do not over-beat.

2. Beat the egg whites with an electric beater until firm peaks form, then gently fold into the ricotta mixture, along with the blueberries.

3. Spray a large nonstick frying pan lightly with oil, and heat over a low heat. Drop ¼ cupfuls of the batter into the pan, and cook for 2 minutes, until golden underneath. Turn and cook a further 1½ minutes, until the hotcakes have risen and are golden brown and cooked through. Repeat with the remaining batter, to make 8 hotcakes. Serve immediately with dollops of yogurt.

SWEET CORN AND MUSHROOM OMELET

Per serving: Calories 286 ■ Protein 22 gFat 17 g (saturated fat 4 g)
Carbohydrate 25 g

GI LOW

Serves 4 ■ Preparation time: 10 minutes ■ Cooking time: 10 minutes

olive oil spray
3½ oz. button mushrooms, sliced
10-oz. can corn kernels, well drained
½ cup flat-leaf parsley, finely chopped
6 eggs
4 slices Shiloh Farms sprouted 7-grain bread, toasted
½ small ripe avocado·

1. Lightly spray a 12-inch nonstick frying pan with olive oil. Cook the mushrooms on low heat for 2 minutes, or until soft.

2. Combine the mushrooms, corn, and parsley in a bowl. In a jug or bowl, whisk 3 of the eggs until lightly beaten. Pour into the frying pan, and cook over a medium heat for 2 minutes, until almost set.

3. Sprinkle half the corn mixture over half of the omelet surface, and fold over to enclose. Cook for a further 2–3 minutes, then cut the omelet in half using a nonscratch spatula. Repeat with remaining ingredients. Spread the toast with avocado and serve with the omelet.

CORN AND ZUCCHINI MUFFINS

These muffins are best eaten on the day they are made.
From The New Glucose Revolution Low GI Vegetarian Cookbook,
page 83

Per serving: Calories402 ■ Protein 16 g ■ Fiber 9 g ■ Fat 13 g (saturated 4
g) Carbohydrate 50 g

GI MEDIUM

Serves 6 ■ Preparation time: 15 minutes ■ Cooking time: 30 minutes
Cooling time: 15 minutes

2 cups stone-ground whole wheat self-rising flour
2 teaspoons baking powder
1½ cups fresh corn kernels (about 3 small cobs)
2 (about 9 oz.) zucchini, finely grated, moisture squeezed out
1 carrot (about 4½ oz.), finely grated
⅓ cup finely grated parmesan
1½ cups buttermilk
2 tablespoons light olive oil
2 eggs

1. Preheat oven to 350 F. Lightly grease a 6-cup large muffin pan.
2. Place the flour, baking powder, corn, zucchini, carrot, and parmesan in a large bowl and mix well. Add to the dry ingredients and mix until just combined.
3. Spoon the mixture evenly among the muffin cups. Bake for 25–30 minutes, or until golden and a skewer inserted into the centers comes out clean. Set aside in the pan for 15 minutes before turning out. Serve warm or at room temperature.

PANCAKES WITH TOFU, BASIL, AND SUN-DRIED TOMATO

From The New Glucose Revolution Low GI Vegetarian Cookbook, *page 86*

Per serving: Calories 417 ■ Protein 22 g ■ Fat 12 g (saturated fat 2 g) Carbohydrate 51 g

GI MEDIUM

Serves 4 (makes 8) ■ Preparation time: 15 minutes
Cooking time: 40 minutes

10½ oz. silken tofu, drained
2 eggs
1 cup low-fat soy milk
1 cup stone-ground whole wheat self-rising flour
½ cup buckwheat flour
1 tablespoon baking powder
½ cup sun-dried tomatoes, patted dry with paper towel, finely chopped
½ cup finely shredded basil
olive oil spray
2¼ oz. baby arugula leaves
½ cup strips grilled red pepper
1 tablespoon balsamic vinegar
1½ teaspoons flaxseed oil
salt and freshly ground black pepper

1. To make the pancakes, place the tofu in a bowl and use a fork to mash. Whisk in the eggs and soy milk. Sift in the whole wheat flour, buckwheat flour, and baking powder until well combined. Stir in the sun-dried tomatoes and basil.

2. Spray a large nonstick frying pan with oil and place over medium heat. Drop ⅓ cup of the batter into the pan, spreading it out to about 6 inches in diameter. Cook for 3 minutes, or until golden underneath. Turn and cook another 2 minutes, or until the pancake has risen and is golden brown and cooked through. Repeat with the remaining batter to make 8 pancakes.

3. Place the arugula and grilled pepper into a bowl. Whisk the vinegar and flaxseed oil together and season. Add to arugula mixture and toss to combine. Divide pancakes among serving plates, top with dressed arugula and pepper, and serve.

Quick-and-Easy Light Meals

(on the table in about 30 minutes)

TUNA AND BEAN SALAD
WITH GARLIC PITA TOASTS

Per serving: Calories 340 ■ Protein 25 g ■ Fat 8 g (saturated fat 1 g)
Carbohydrate 36 g

GI LOW

Serves 4 ■ Preparation time: 10 minutes ■ Cooking time: 2–3 minutes

6-oz. can of light tuna, drained and flaked
1 small red onion, very finely sliced
2 ripe tomatoes, cut into thin wedges
13-oz. can of cannellini beans, rinsed and drained
1 bunch arugula, trimmed and leaves torn
2 tablespoons lemon juice
1 tablespoon extra-virgin olive oil
salt and freshly ground black pepper, to taste
4 small 100% whole wheat pita breads
1 large garlic clove, peeled and halved

1. Combine the tuna, onion, tomatoes, beans, and arugula in a large bowl. Drizzle with lemon juice and olive oil, season with salt and pepper, and toss gently to combine.
2. Toast the pita bread on both sides, then rub the cut garlic clove all over one side. Break into pieces, and serve with the salad.

BEAN AND CORN BURRITOS

This makes a delicious lunch to take to work. Store the bean mixture in an airtight container, and the lettuce and cheese in another. One option is to use whole wheat lavash bread in place of the tortillas, then assemble just before eating.

Per serving: Calories 434 ■ Protein 21 g ■ Fat 12 g (saturated fat 4.5 g)
Carbohydrate 60 g

GI LOW

Serves 4 ■ Preparation time: 10 minutes ■ Cooking time: 5 minutes

13 oz. corn kernels, drained
13 oz. red kidney beans, rinsed and drained
2 large ripe tomatoes, chopped
2 shallots, finely sliced
⅓ cup taco sauce
6-inch white corn tortillas
4 large iceberg lettuce leaves, shredded
¾ cup reduced-fat cheese, grated

1. Preheat the oven to 350°F.
2. Combine the corn, beans, tomatoes, shallots, and taco sauce in a bowl.
3. Wrap the tortillas in foil and warm in the oven for 5 minutes.
4. To assemble, spread a lettuce leaf over a warmed tortilla, and top with the bean mixture and grated cheese. Fold the bottom of the tortilla over the filling, and roll up to enclose. Serve immediately.

GRILLED BEEF WITH THAI NOODLE SALAD

Per serving: Calories 267 ■ Protein 31 g ■ Fat 11.5 g (saturated fat 3.5 g)
Carbohydrate 9 g

GI LOW

Serves 4 ■ Preparation time: 25 minutes ■ Cooking time: 10 minutes

2 oz. rice vermicelli, dry
1 carrot, peeled and cut into thin strips
1 cucumber, cut into thin strips
1 red pepper, cut into thin strips
2 cups bean sprouts
1 bunch mint, leaves picked and torn
1 bunch coriander, leaves only
1 ½ tablespoons lime juice
1 tablespoon fish sauce
1 tablespoon peanut oil
1 teaspoon granulated sugar
1 small fresh red chili, finely chopped
4 beef tenderloin steaks, trimmed of excess fat (about 4½ oz. each)
1 teaspoon peanut oil, extra
freshly ground black pepper, to taste

1. Place the rice vermicelli in a bowl and cover with plenty of cold water. Set aside for 5 minutes, or until the noodles become translucent. Drain well and cut into short lengths.

2. Place the vermicelli, carrot, cucumber, pepper, bean sprouts, mint, and coriander in a large serving bowl. Toss well to combine.

3. Whisk the lime juice, fish sauce, peanut oil, sugar, and chili together.

4. Preheat a grill on medium-high. If you don't have a grill you can use a heavy-based frying pan. Brush the steaks with the extra peanut oil and season with pepper. Cook, turning frequently, for 10 minutes, or until a thermometer inserted in the center of the steak registers 160°F for medium. Set aside for 5 minutes.

5. Add the dressing to the salad and toss to coat. Serve the noodle salad with the steaks.

GRILLED FISH WITH WHITE BEAN SALSA

This white bean salsa can be made ahead of time and kept in the refrigerator until you are ready to serve. For a change, try it with grilled chicken, or as a light meal on its own with Alvarado Street Bakery 100% sprouted sourdough bread.

Per serving: Calories 273 ■ Protein 33 g ■ Fat 17.5 g (saturated fat 2.5 g) Carbohydrate 11 g

GI LOW

Serves 4 ■ Preparation time: 15 minutes ■ Cooking time: 10 minutes

4 3½-oz. firm white-fleshed fish cutlets, such as cod or halibut
1 teaspoon olive oil

WHITE BEAN SALSA

13 oz. white beans, rinsed and drained
2 ripe tomatoes, finely chopped
3 shallots, thinly sliced
⅓ cup fresh coriander leaves, shredded
1½ tablespoons fresh lime juice
1 tablespoon extra-virgin olive oil
salt and freshly ground black pepper, to taste

To Serve
4 cups mixed salad leaves (mesclun)
2 tablespoons vinaigrette dressing (see recipe below)

1. To make the salsa, place the beans, tomatoes, shallots, coriander, lime juice, and olive oil in a small bowl and toss lightly to combine. Season well with salt and pepper and set aside while you prepare the fish.

2. Preheat a grill on medium-high. If you don't have a grill, use a heavy-based frying pan.

3. Brush both sides of the fish with olive oil and season with salt
   and pepper. Grill the fish for 4 minutes on each side, or until the
   fish is opaque and flakes gently when tested with a fork. Serve
   with the salsa, salad, and a light vinaigrette dressing.

Cook's tip: Mesclun is simply a mix of fresh, tender young salad leaves and
may include a variety of lettuces such as iceberg, Romaine, mignonette, and
oakleaf, plus baby spinach leaves, arugula, curly endive, broadleaf endive, nas-
turtium, snow pea shoots, radicchio, and sometimes edible flowers. You can
buy it ready-made in most supermarkets, or mix your own to taste.

VINAIGRETTE DRESSING

In a screw-top jar combine 2 tablespoons olive oil with the juice
of 1 lemon, 1 tablespoon of white wine vinegar, a clove of crushed
garlic, and one teaspoon of grainy mustard. Add 1 tablespoon of
finely chopped flat-leaf parsley, 1 small tomato that has been very
finely diced, and 3 to 4 finely diced pitted black olives. Shake to
combine. Stand about 30 minutes before serving.

Serves 8

TOMATO FETTUCINE WITH SALMON AND BABY SPINACH

Per serving: Calories 476 ■ Protein 33 g ■ Fat 15.5 g (saturated fat 6.5 g)
Carbohydrate 45 g

GI LOW

Serves 4 ■ Preparation time: 10 minutes ■ Cooking time: 10 minutes

3 teaspoons extra-virgin olive oil
1 large red onion, cut into thin wedges
⅓ cup capers, drained and patted dry with paper towel
2 cloves garlic, crushed
4 large ripe tomatoes, chopped
⅓ cup vegetable stock
1 lb. fresh fettuccine
4 cups baby spinach leaves
2 7-oz. cans red salmon, bones and skin removed, broken into large pieces
2 tablespoons fresh lemon juice
salt and freshly ground black pepper, to taste

1. Heat the oil in a large frying pan over medium heat. Add the onion, capers, and garlic and cook, stirring often, for 6–7 minutes or until the onion softens. Add the tomatoes and stir for 1 minute. Add the stock and increase the heat to high. Bring to the boil then remove from the heat.

2. Meanwhile, cook the pasta in a large saucepan of salted water for 2–3 minutes or until tender. Drain well and return to the pan.

3. Add the onion mixture and spinach leaves to the pasta. Toss well until combined and the spinach starts to wilt. Add the salmon and lemon juice. Toss gently and season to taste. Serve immediately.

Cook's tip: Most types of pasta have a similar GI, so spaghetti or fusilli, for example, could also be used in this recipe.

PORK WITH CREAMY MUSTARD SAUCE

Per serving: Calories 311 ■ Protein 41 g ■ Fat 9 g (saturated fat 2 g)
Carbohydrate 17 g

GI LOW

Serves 4 ■ Preparation time: 10 minutes ■ Cooking time: 20 minutes

1 tablespoon olive oil
5 cups (about ½ large head) red cabbage, thinly sliced
2 carrots, grated
1 yellow onion, cut into thin wedges
½ cup chicken stock
4 pork cutlets (about 5¼ oz. each), trimmed of excess fat
1 cup orange juice
½ cup light evaporated milk
1 tablespoon whole-grain mustard
¼ cup chopped fresh dill
salt and freshly ground black pepper, to taste

1. Heat half the oil in a large, heavy-based saucepan over medium heat. Add the cabbage, carrots, and onion. Cook, stirring, for 3 minutes. Add the stock, cover, and reduce the heat to low. Cook for 15 minutes, or until the vegetables are tender.

2. Meanwhile, heat the remaining oil in a large, heavy-based frying pan over medium heat. Add the pork cutlets and cook for 4–6 minutes on each side, or until lightly browned and no longer pink in the center. Transfer to a plate, cover loosely with foil, and set aside.

3. Increase the pan heat to high and add the orange juice, evaporated milk, and mustard. Bring to the boil, stirring. Boil uncovered for 6–7 minutes, stirring often, until the sauce reduces and thickens slightly. Return the cutlets to the pan and turn to coat in the sauce.

4. Stir the dill into the cabbage mixture and season well. To serve, spoon the sauce over the cutlets and accompany with the vegetables.

TOFU AND VEGETABLE NOODLES

Per serving: Calories 381 ■ Protein 19 g ■ Fat 14 g (saturated fat 1.5 g)
Carbohydrate 44 g

GI LOW

Serves 4 ■ Preparation time: 10 minutes (plus 4 hours for marinating)
Cooking time: 15 minutes

⅓ cup soy sauce

¼ cup oyster sauce

¼ cup hoisin sauce

2 cloves garlic, crushed

14 oz. firm tofu, drained and cut into 1-inch pieces

1 lb. Hokkien noodles

1½ tablespoons olive oil

1 yellow onion, cut into thin wedges

1 red bell pepper, cut into thin strips

7 oz. baby eggplant, thinly sliced lengthways

8-oz. can bamboo shoot slices, drained

2 tablespoons water

1. Combine the soy, oyster, and hoisin sauce with the garlic in a shallow glass dish. Add the tofu and turn to coat in the marinade. Cover and refrigerate for 4 hours, turning once.

2. Place the noodles in a large heatproof bowl and cover with boiling water. Set aside for 5 minutes then drain well.

3. Heat 2 teaspoons of the oil in a wok over a high heat. Add the onion, bell pepper, and eggplant. Stir-fry for 2–3 minutes, or until the vegetables are almost tender. Toss in the bamboo shoots. Add the water, cover, and cook for 1–2 minutes. Transfer the vegetables to a bowl.

4. Wipe out the wok. Add the remaining oil and heat over high heat. Drain the tofu, reserving the marinade. Stir-fry the tofu for 2–3 minutes, or until golden. Return the vegetables to the wok and add the reserved marinade and noodles. Toss for 1–2 minutes, or until well combined and heated through. Serve immediately.

CHICKPEA AND BEET SALAD

Per serving: Calories 395 ■ Protein 20 g ■ Fat 11.5 g (saturated fat 1.5 g)
Carbohydrate 54 g

GI LOW

Serves 4 ■ Preparation time: 20 minutes

2 14½-oz. cans chickpeas, rinsed and drained
1 red onion, cut into thin wedges
4 cups baby arugula leaves
1 tablespoon extra-virgin olive oil
1½ tablespoons lemon juice
1 clove garlic, crushed
pinch granulated sugar, salt, and freshly ground black pepper, to taste
16-oz. can beet wedges, drained and patted dry with paper towel
4 slices Pepperidge Farm Sprouted Wheat bread

1. Place the chickpeas, onion, and arugula in a large serving bowl.
2. Whisk the olive oil, vinegar, lemon juice, garlic, and sugar. Season with salt and pepper.
3. Add the dressing to the salad and toss gently to combine. Then add the beetroot and toss gently again. Serve with the bread.

PISTACHIO AND QUINOA TABBOULEH

Quinoa is a tiny, fast-cooking grain ideal in gluten-free dishes. It's not just low GI—it's also rich in nutrients, including protein. Enjoy this tabbouleh on its own, in iceberg lettuce-leaf scoops, in gluten-free wraps or pita pockets with hummus, or as a salad accompaniment to a barbecue. Store leftover salad in an airtight container in the refrigerator for up to 1 day.

From The New Glucose Revolution Low GI Gluten-Free Eating Made Easy, *page 150*

Per serving (of tabbouleh only): Calories 275 ■ Protein 8 g ■ Fiber 5.5 g
Fat 14 g (saturated fat 1.5 g) ■ Carbohydrate 25 g

GI LOW

Serves 6 ■ Preparation time: 10 minutes
Cooking time: 15 minutes + resting time

To Serve

1 cup quinoa, rinsed

juice of 1 lemon, or to taste

2½ tablespoons extra-virgin olive oil

freshly ground black pepper

½ cup roughly chopped pistachio nuts

1 cup chopped flat-leaf (Italian) parsley

½ cup chopped mint leaves, or to taste

1 small red (Spanish) onion, finely diced

2 large vine-ripened tomatoes, deseeded and chopped

1 medium Lebanese cucumber, deseeded and diced

gluten-free wraps

hummus

1. Place the quinoa in a medium saucepan and cover with 2 cups of water. Bring to a boil, then reduce the heat and simmer for 10–15 minutes or until the grains are just tender and translucent and all the water is absorbed. Remove from the heat and let rest, covered, for 5–10 minutes. Fluff with a fork.

2. Meanwhile, whisk together the lemon juice and oil and season to taste.

3. Transfer the warm quinoa to a serving bowl with the nuts, parsley, mint, onion, tomato, cucumber, and dressing. Mix well to combine. Serve in a bowl, or with gluten-free wraps and hummus, to scoop and wrap your salad if you like.

Variation: For an even more colorful salad, use red quinoa (you'll find it in health food stores) and follow the cooking times suggested on the package.

INDIVIDUAL FRITTATAS WITH PEPPER, SWEET POTATO, BABY PEAS, AND FETA

From The New Glucose Revolution Low GI Vegetarian Cookbook, *page 100*

Per serving: Calories 251 ■ Protein 17 g ■ Fiber 5 g
Fat 12 g (saturated 4 g) ■ Carbohydrate 16 g

GI MEDIUM

Serves 6 ■ Preparation time: 15 minutes ■ Cooking time: 30–35 minutes
Cooling time: 10 minutes

1 tablespoon extra-virgin olive oil

1 red onion, halved, thinly sliced

1 red pepper, cut into short, thin strips

10½ oz. orange sweet potato, cut into ½-inch pieces

1 clove garlic, crushed

1 cup frozen baby green peas

⅓ cup semi-dried tomatoes, finely chopped

3½ oz. low fat feta, crumbled

olive oil spray

7 eggs

½ cup low fat-milk or soy milk

salt and freshly ground black pepper

1. Heat the oil in a large, nonstick frying pan over medium-high heat. Add the onion, pepper, sweet potato, and garlic. Cook, stirring often, for 5 minutes. Add the peas and cook for 3 minutes. Remove from the heat and set aside to cool a little. Stir in the semi-dried tomatoes and feta.

2. Preheat oven to 375 F. Spray a large 6–cup muffin pan with oil. Whisk together the eggs and milk, and season. Divide the vegetables among the muffin pan cups. Pour the egg mixture evenly over the vegetables.

3. Bake for 20–25 minutes, or until the frittatas are set and lightly golden. Set aside in the pan for 10 minutes before turning out. Serve warm with dressed salad leaves.

CARAMELIZED ONION AND GOAT CHEESE PIZZA, AND GRILLED VEGETABLE PIZZA

From The New Glucose Revolution Low GI Vegetarian Cookbook, *page 109*

Per serving:
Caramelized onion and goat cheese: Calories 293 ■ Protein 9 g ■ Fiber 7 g
■ Fat 12 g (saturated 3 g) ■ Carbohydrate 34 g

GI MEDIUM

Grilled vegetable: Calories 375 ■ Protein 17 g ■ Fiber 10 g
Fat 14 g (saturated 5 g) ■ Carbohydrate 40 g

GI MEDIUM

Serves 4 ■ Preparation time: 20 minutes ■ Standing time: 1 hour
Cooking time: 40–50 minutes

1½ cups stone-ground whole wheat all-purpose flour
¼-oz. sachet dried yeast
1 teaspoon salt

Caramelized onion and goat cheese topping
2 tablespoons olive oil
1 lb 10 oz. red onions, halved, thinly sliced
2 tablespoons fresh thyme leaves
2 cloves garlic, crushed
1 tablespoon brown sugar
1 tablespoon balsamic vinegar
2¼ oz. goat cheese, crumbled

Grilled vegetable topping
2 tablespoons basil pesto
3½ oz. grilled red pepper, patted dry with paper towel, cut into thin strips
2½ oz. drained marinated artichoke hearts, cut into thin wedges
2½ oz. grilled eggplant, patted dry with paper towel, cut into thin strips
2¼ oz. bocconcini, thinly sliced
¼ fresh basil leaves, to serve

1. To make the pizza dough, place the flour, yeast, and salt in a bowl. Add ¾ cup lukewarm water and use a flat-bladed knife to mix until just combined. Turn out onto a lightly floured surface and knead until smooth. Place in a lightly oiled bowl, cover with plastic wrap, and set aside in a warm place for 1 hour.

2. Meanwhile, to make the caramelized onions, heat the oil in a large nonstick frying pan over medium heat. Add the onion, thyme, and garlic, and stir to coat. Reduce heat to medium-low and cook, stirring occasionally, for 25–30 minutes, or until the onions are very soft. Cook for another 5 minutes or until the onions start to caramelize. Set aside to cool completely.

3. Preheat oven to 450 F. Lightly grease two 11-inch round pizza trays.

4. Use your fist to pound the dough. Divide into two. Roll one portion out and use it to line one tray. Repeat with the remaining dough. Spread the caramelized onions over one of the bases, and sprinkle over the goat cheese. Spread the second base with the pesto. Top with the pepper, artichoke, eggplant, and bocconcini.

5. Bake the pizzas, turning the trays halfway through cooking, for 15–20 minutes, or until the tops are golden and the bases are crisp. Sprinkle the grilled vegetable pizza with basil leaves before serving.

Main Meals

To take a little time over . . .

STUFFED VEGETABLES

You could substitute the pearl barley and quinoa with cooked brown rice or couscous. Any variety of fresh herbs, vegetables, nuts, and seeds can be added to the stuffing mix.

From The New Glucose Revolution Low GI Vegetarian Cookbook, *page 133*

Per serving: Calories 368 ▪ Protein 12 g ▪ Fiber 13 g
Fat 19 g (saturated 2 g) ▪ Carbohydrate 31g

GI LOW

Serves 4 ▪ Preparation time: 25 minutes ▪ Cooking time: 1 hour

½ *cup pearl barley*
⅓ *cup quinoa*
2 medium-sized eggplants, halved lengthwise
6 large vine-ripened tomatoes
1 tablespoon olive oil
1 onion, finely chopped
1 stick celery, chopped
2 cloves garlic, crushed
2 teaspoons ground cumin
1 teaspoon dried oregano
1 zucchini, finely chopped
¼ *cup pine nuts*
¼ *cup pumpkin seeds*
2 tablespoons freshly chopped mint
2 tablespoons freshly chopped parsley
finely grated zest of 1 lemon
salt and freshly ground black pepper
2 red peppers, halved lengthwise, deseeded

1. Place the pearl barley, quinoa, and 3 cups water in a medium-sized saucepan. Bring to the boil, then cover and simmer for 30 minutes or until grains are tender. Drain well.

2. Meanwhile, scoop out the flesh of the eggplants, leaving a ½-inch-thick shell. Sprinkle the insides with salt and place upside down on a paper towel to drain off the bitter juices. Dice the flesh.

3. Preheat oven to 350 F. Deseed and dice 2 of the tomatoes. Cut the tops off the remaining 4 tomatoes and scoop out their seeds, leaving a shell. Set aside.

4. Heat the oil in a large frying pan over medium-low heat. Add the onion and celery and cook, stirring occasionally, for 5 minutes, or until vegetables are soft. Add the garlic, cumin, oregano, and zucchini and cook, stirring, for 1 minute. Increase the heat to medium-high, add the chopped eggplant and zucchini and cook, stirring for 2–3 minutes, or until lightly golden. Add the drained barley and quinoa, the chopped tomato, pine nuts, pumpkin seeds, mint, parsley, and lemon zest, and season.

5. Rinse out the eggplant shells and pat dry. Fill the eggplants, tomatoes, and peppers with the stuffing mixture, place on a lightly oiled baking tray and roast for 30 minutes, or until vegetables are soft and golden brown. Serve.

SHIITAKE GINGER AND TOFU HOKKIEN NOODLES

Chinese black vinegar is available from Asian supermarkets. It's a delicious addition to Asian stir-fries, marinades, and salad dressings.
From The New Glucose Revolution Low GI Vegetarian Cookbook, *page 139*

Per serving: Calories 390 ■ Protein 20 g ■ Fiber 8 g
Fat 12 g (saturated 2 g) ■ Carbohydrate 4g

GI LOW

Serves 4 ■ Preparation time: 15 minutes ■ Marinating time: 4 hours
Cooking time: 10 minutes

2 tablespoons soy sauce
2 tablespoons Chinese rice wine
1 tablespoon Chinese black vinegar
1 clove garlic, crushed
2 teaspoons finely grated ginger
1 13-oz. package firm tofu, cut into 5/8 cubes
1 lb package Hokkien noodles
1 tablespoon olive oil
1 ¼-inch piece ginger, cut into very thin matchsticks
1 long red chile, deseeded, thinly sliced
5½ oz. baby corn, halved lengthwise
5½ oz. fresh shiitake mushrooms, halved
5½ oz. sugar snap peas, strings removed
6 scallions, trimmed, cut into 1 ½ inch lengths
1 bunch bok choy, trimmed, cut into equal lengths

1. Combine the soy sauce, rice wine, vinegar, garlic, and grated ginger in a shallow, non-metallic dish. Add the tofu and turn to coat in the marinade. Cover and refrigerate for 4 hours, turning once.

2. Meanwhile, place the noodles in a large heatproof bowl and cover with boiling water. Set aside for 5 minutes, then drain well.

3. Heat half the oil in a large wok or frying pan. With a slotted spoon add the tofu (reserving the marinade) in batches and fry until golden. Remove and set aside.

4. Heat the remaining oil, add the sliced ginger and chile and stir-fry for 30 seconds. Add the baby corn and mushrooms and stir-fry for 2 minutes more. Add the sugar snap peas and scallion and cook for 1 minute, then add the bok choy and reserved marinade. Toss together for 1–2 minutes over heat. Return the tofu to the wok and toss to combine and heat through.

5. Place the noodles in the bowls and top with the vegetables and marinade liquid.

3-BEAN CHILI WITH SPICY TORTILLA CRISPS

Guacamole goes particularly well with this recipe.
From The New Glucose Revolution Low GI Vegetarian Cookbook,
page 136

Per serving: Calories 296 ■ Protein 14 g ■ Fiber 14 g
Fat 7 g (saturated 1 g) ■ Carbohydrate 38 g

GI LOW

Serves 4 ■ Preparation time: 20 minutes ■ Soaking time: overnight
Cooking time: 50 minutes

1 tablespoon olive oil
1 onion, finely chopped
1 carrot, peeled, finely chopped
1 stick celery, finely chopped
2 cloves garlic, crushed
1 long red chile, finely chopped
½ teaspoon chile powder
½ teaspoon dried oregano
1 small red pepper, deseeded, finely chopped
1 small green pepper, deseeded, finely chopped
2 small zucchini, sliced
2 tablespoons tomato paste
1 14-oz. can red kidney beans, rinsed and drained
½ cup black-eyed peas, soaked overnight
salt and freshly ground black pepper
juice of 1 lime
2 tablespoons chopped cilantro
spicy tortilla chips
4 purchased corn tortillas
olive oil spray
½ teaspoon paprika
¼ teaspoon chile powder

1. Heat the oil in a large heavy-based saucepan over medium-low
   heat. Add the onion, carrot, and celery and cook, stirring occasionally, for 6–7 minutes, or until the vegetables are slightly soft.
   Add the garlic, chile, chile powder, and oregano and cook,
   stirring, for 1–2 minutes, or until fragrant. Add the pepper and
   zucchini and cook for 1 minute more.

2. Add the tomato paste and cook, stirring, for 1 minute. Add the chopped tomatoes and stock, and stir to combine. Add the bulgur and beans. Bring to a boil, then reduce the heat to very low and simmer, covered, stirring frequently, for 30 minutes or until beans and vegetables are tender.

3. Season, add lime juice to taste, and mix in the chopped cilantro.

4. To make the Spicy Tortilla Chips, preheat oven to 350 F. Spray both sides of each tortilla lightly with olive oil. Sprinkle with the paprika and chile powder. Place the tortillas on a large baking tray and bake in the oven for 5–6 minutes, or until crisp. Cut into quarters and serve with the chili.

Cook's tip: You can use any spices on the tortillas, such as ground coriander, cumin, or cayenne pepper.

FENNEL, LEEK, AND BEAN BARLEY PILAF

Both fennel and fennel seeds have been added to this dish for extra flavor. Any variety of vegetables can be used.

From The New Glucose Revolution Low GI Vegetarian Cookbook, *page 113*

Per serving: Calories 319 ▪ Protein 11g ▪ Fiber 11 g
Fat 11 g (saturated 1 g) ▪ Carbohydrate 39 g

GI LOW

Serves 4 ▪ Preparation time: 15 minutes ▪ Cooking time: 50 minutes

1 tablespoon olive oil
1 leek, trimmed and finely chopped
1 small fennel bulb, trimmed, finely chopped
1 clove garlic, crushed
½ teaspoon fennel seeds, lightly toasted, crushed
4 oz. button mushrooms, sliced
1 corn cob, kernels removed
1 cup pearl barley
2 cups hot vegetable stock
5½ oz. green beans, trimmed, sliced
salt and freshly ground black pepper
2 tablespoons chopped parsley
¼ cup slivered almonds, lightly toasted, to serve

1. Heat the oil in a large heavy-based saucepan, add the leek and fennel and cook over medium-low heat, sitting occasionally, for 6–7 minutes, or until leek is soft. Add the garlic and fennel seeds and cook, stirring, for 1 minute more.

2. Increase the heat to medium-high. Add the mushrooms and corn and cook, stirring, for 2 minutes. Add the barley and stock, stir to combine, and bring to a boil. Reduce the heat to low, cover and simmer, stirring occasionally, for 35–40 minutes or until the barley is almost tender and the stock absorbed.

3. Add the green beans and season, cook for 3 minutes more, then mix in the parsley. Serve sprinkled with the almonds.

VEGETARIAN PAELLA

Paella makes a fantastic addition to a party menu. It is easy to prepare, as it is all cooked in one pan. You can add practically anything you like.
   From The New Glucose Revolution Low GI Vegetarian Cookbook, *page 129*

Per serving: Calories 361 ■ Protein 15 g ■ Fiber 6 g
Fat 12 g (saturated 2 g) ■ Carbohydrate 45 g

GI MEDIUM

Serves 6–8 ■ Preparation time: 20 minutes ■ Cooking time: 35 minutes

1 tablespoon olive oil
2 red onions, thinly sliced
2 cloves garlic, crushed
1 teaspoon sweet smoked paprika
2 teaspoons paprika
10½ oz. basmati rice
½ teaspoon saffron strands
4 cups good-quality vegetable stock
1 red pepper roasted, peeled, sliced
1 green pepper, roasted, peeled, sliced
2 vine-ripened tomatoes, deseeded, chopped
¾ cup fresh corn kernels (about 1 large cob)
1 cup frozen baby peas, thawed
10½ oz. firm tofu, cut into ¾ chunks
6 oz. drained marinated artichoke hearts, cut into thin wedges
⅓ cup pine nuts, lightly toasted, to serve

1. Heat the oil in a large, heavy-based saucepan over medium-low heat. Add the onion and cook, stirring occasionally, for 5–6 minutes or until the onion is soft. Add the garlic and cook, stirring, for 1 minute. Add the paprikas and cook, stirring, for 1 minute more. Add the rice and stir to coat the grains in the spices.

2. Add the saffron to the vegetable stock, then add the stock to the rice. Bring to a boil, then reduce heat to low, cover the pan with a lid or a piece of foil and simmer for 20–25 minutes, or until the stock is absorbed and the rice is cooked.

3. Add the peppers, tomato, corn, peas, and tofu, stir to combine, cover and again and cook for another 5 minutes. Remove from the heat and mix in the artichokes. Serve garnished with the pine nuts.

PASTA WITH
ROASTED VEGETABLES AND FETA

Per serving: Calories 393 ■ Protein 18 g
Fat 6 g (saturated fat 2.5 g) ■ Carbohydrate 65 g

GI LOW

Serves 4 ■ Preparation time: 20 minutes ■ Cooking time: 45 minutes

1 small red onion, peeled and cut into wedges
1 red bell pepper, cut into 1¼-inch pieces
2 Roma tomatoes, quartered lengthways
6½ oz. sweet potato, peeled and cut into ¾-inch chunks
1 small eggplant, cut into ¾-inch chunks
olive oil spray
10 oz. short pasta, such as penne or spirals
3½ oz. reduced-fat feta, crumbled
¼ cup basil leaves, shredded
1 small garlic clove, crushed (optional)

1. Preheat the oven to 350°F.

2. Spread the onion, bell pepper, tomatoes, sweet potato, and eggplant on two large oven trays, spray lightly with oil, and toss the vegetables to coat. Roast for about 45 minutes, until tender and browned.

3. When the vegetables are almost ready, cook the pasta in a large saucepan of boiling water, according to the packet directions, until al dente. Drain well and return to the pan. Add the vegetables, feta, basil, and garlic and toss to combine. Serve immediately.

LAMB CUTLETS WITH PEA PILAF

Per serving: Calories 420 ■ Protein 43 g
Fat 12.5 g (saturated fat 4.5 g) ■ Carbohydrate 34 g

GI MEDIUM

Serves 4 ■ Preparation time: 15 minutes (plus 1 hour for marinating)
Cooking time: 30 minutes

½ cup plain low-fat yogurt
1 teaspoon ground coriander
1 teaspoon ground cumin
2 teaspoons freshly grated ginger
8 lean lamb cutlets

PEA PILAF

2 teaspoons canola oil
1 small onion, halved and sliced
4 cardamom pods, lightly crushed
½ teaspoon ground turmeric
⅔ cup basmati rice
7 oz. cauliflower (½ small head), cut into small florets
1 cup vegetable stock
1 head broccoli (about 12 oz.), cut into small florets
1 cup fresh or frozen green peas

1. Combine the yogurt with the coriander, cumin, and ginger. Place the lamb cutlets in a nonmetallic dish and spread the yogurt mixture over the meat section of the cutlets. Cover and refrigerate for 1 hour.

2. To make the pilaf, heat the oil in a large saucepan, and add the onion. Cook over medium heat for 3–5 minutes, stirring often, until the onion is soft and lightly golden. Add the cardamom pods, turmeric, and rice, and cook, stirring, for 30 seconds.

3. Add the cauliflower and stock, stir once, then cover and bring to the boil. Reduce the heat to very low, and cook tightly covered for 10 minutes. Add the broccoli and peas and cook for a further 10 minutes. Remove from the heat and stand, still covered, for five minutes.

4. Meanwhile, heat a grill or nonstick frying pan, and cook the lamb over medium-high heat for 4–6 minutes on each side, or until lightly browned and no longer pink in the center. Serve the lamb cutlets with the rice pilaf.

LENTIL AND RICOTTA CANNELLONI

Per serving: Calories 339 ■ Protein 25 g ■ Fat 11.5 g (saturated fat 5.7 g)
Carbohydrate 33 g

GI LOW

Serves 6 ■ Preparation time: 30 minutes ■ Cooking time: 1 hour

2 teaspoons olive oil

1 small onion, finely chopped

2 garlic cloves, crushed

14-oz. can chopped tomatoes

1 cup vegetable stock

1 cup red lentils

1 bunch spinach, raw, stems trimmed

salt and freshly ground black pepper, to taste

4 fresh lasagna sheets (6 x 12 inches)

1¾ cups reduced-fat fresh ricotta

pinch nutmeg

2 cups Italian tomato cooking sauce

½ cup grated reduced-fat cheddar cheese

1. Preheat the oven to 400°F.

2. Heat the oil in a large saucepan, and cook the onion over a low heat for 5 minutes, until soft. Add the garlic and stir for a further 30 seconds, then add the tomatoes, stock, and lentils. Bring to the boil, reduce the heat to low, and simmer for 20 minutes, covered, until the lentils are tender. Stir occasionally to prevent the mixture from catching on the bottom of the pan.

3. Roughly chop the spinach leaves and stir into the lentil mixture to wilt. Season the mixture with salt and pepper, then cool to room temperature.

4. Meanwhile, cut each lasagna sheet crossways into three pieces. Mash the ricotta in a bowl with the nutmeg until smooth. Then spread 1 cup of the tomato sauce over the base of a large lasagna dish.

5. Spread ¼ cup of the lentil mixture along the center of a lasagna piece. Spoon 1 heaping tablespoon of ricotta over the lentil mixture. Roll up to enclose, and place seam side down in the lasagna dish. Repeat with the remaining ingredients, fitting them snugly into the dish. Pour the remaining tomato sauce over to cover, and sprinkle with cheese.

6. Bake for 35 minutes, until the pasta is tender. Serve with a green salad.

GRILLED LEMON CHICKEN SKEWERS

We've allowed an hour to marinate the chicken, but if you have the time, leave it a little longer to absorb the flavors of the marinade. The skewer enters the meat 3–4 times, like a needle threading through cloth.

From The New Glucose Revolution Low GI Gluten-Free Eating Made Easy, *page 172*

Per serving (without salad): Calories 485 ■ Protein 38 g ■ Fiber 2.5 g
Fat 16 g (saturated fat 3.5 g) ■ Carbohydrates 46 g

GI MEDIUM

Serves 4 ■ Preparation time: 25 minutes ■ Marinating time: 1 hour
Cooking time: 30 minutes + standing time

21 oz. skinless, boneless chicken breasts (2 large)

Marinade
1 teaspoon finely grated lemon rind
½ cup lemon juice
1 teaspoon chopped fresh rosemary
1 tablespoon Dijon mustard
2 cloves garlic, crushed
1½ tablespoons olive oil

Bean and Asparagus Pilaf
1 bunch asparagus, cut into 1-inch pieces
4 oz. (about 12) green beans, trimmed and cut into 1-inch pieces
2 teaspoons olive oil
1 onion, chopped
1 clove garlic, crushed
1 cup basmati rice
2 cups gluten-free, reduced-salt chicken stock
2½ tablespoons chopped parsley

To Serve
green salad with vinaigrette dressing

1. Soak 12 wooden skewers in water for 30 minutes.

2. Meanwhile, slice each chicken breast into 6-by-½-inch-thick long slices. You should have 12 long slices. Place 4 pieces on a sheet of plastic wrap, and cover with another sheet of plastic wrap. Use a rolling pin or mallet to flatten the pieces to about ¼-inch thick. Repeat with the remaining slices.

3. To make the marinade, combine all the ingredients in a medium bowl. Reserve ¼ cup of the mixture and set aside.

4. Add the chicken to remaining marinade in the bowl and chill in the refrigerator for 1 hour.

5. Meanwhile, to make the pilaf, steam the asparagus and beans for 2–3 minutes or until tender. Drain, rinse under cold water, and set aside.

6. Heat the oil in a medium saucepan. Add the onion and cook for 3–4 minutes or until soft and golden. Add the garlic and rice, and cook for 1 more minute, stirring. Add the stock, bring to a boil, then reduce the heat to low and simmer, covered, for 15 minutes. Let stand for 5 minutes. Stir through the beans, asparagus, parsley, and reserved marinade. Set aside, keeping warm.

7. Thread the chicken onto the skewers. Heat the grill and cook chicken each side for 2 minutes or until golden and cooked through.

8. To serve, spoon about ½ cup pilaf onto each plate, top with chicken, and serve with the salad.

CHICKEN MANGO RICE PAPER ROLLS

From The New Glucose Revolution Low GI Gluten-Free Eating Made Easy, *pages 132–136*

Per serving (per roll with dipping sauce): Calories 75 ■ Protein 6 g ■ Fiber 0.5 g ■ Fat 1 g (saturated fat 0.5 g) ■ Carbohydrate 10 g

GI LOW

Serves 12 ■ Preparation time: 30 minutes ■ Cooking time: 10 minutes

1 (9-oz.) chicken breast
2 oz. bean thread noodles
1 mango, peeled and cut into short strips
2 oz. (about 6) snow peas, trimmed and sliced diagonally in half
¼ cup shredded mint
12 round 8-inch rice papers

Dipping Sauce
⅓ cup lime juice
1½ tablespoons fish sauce
1½ tablespoons superfine sugar

1. Put about 1½ cups water in a small saucepan (enough to cover the chicken) and bring to a boil. Add the chicken, reduce the heat, and simmer, covered, for 10 minutes. Set aside to cool in the pan. When chicken is cool enough to handle, shred and then refrigerate.

2. Place the noodles in a heatproof bowl and cover with boiling water. Leave for 3–4 minutes or until soft, then drain. Rinse the noodles under running water to cool, drain again, and cut into short lengths (½–1 inch).

3. To make the dipping sauce, combine all ingredients in a bowl and stir until sugar dissolves. Set aside.

4. Place all filling ingredients on a counter. Dip the wrappers one at a time in a shallow bowl of warm water for 10–15 seconds or until just soft. Drain off excess water and place on a clean surface.

5. Place about 1 tablespoon shredded chicken, 1 heaping teaspoon noodles, 2 strips mango, 2 pieces snow pea, and 1 teaspoon mint on the rice paper, about 1 inch in from the base of the wrapper. Fold up the bottom of the wrapper, then fold in the sides and roll up to enclose the filling. Place on a tray and cover with paper towels. Continue with remaining filling and wrappers.

6. Serve the rolls on a platter with the dipping sauce.

CARROT, AVOCADO, AND SNOW PEA RICE PAPER ROLLS

Squeeze some lime juice over the avocado after it has been sliced to prevent it from turning brown.

From The New Glucose Revolution Low GI Gluten-Free Eating Made Easy, *pages 132–136*

Per serving (per roll with dipping sauce): Calories 86 ▪ Protein 2 g
Fiber 1 g ▪ Fat 5 g (saturated fat 1 g) ▪ Carbohydrate 8 g

GI LOW

Serves 12 ▪ Preparation time: 30 minutes

2 oz. bean thread noodles
1 small carrot, cut into short, thin sticks
1 avocado, cut into short, thin slices
squeeze of lime juice for the avocado
½ bunch garlic chives, cut into 3
2 oz. (about 6) snow peas,
    sliced diagonally in half
2 oz. snow pea sprouts, ends trimmed
12 round 8-inch rice papers

Dipping Sauce
¼ cup gluten-free sweet chili sauce
¼ cup lime juice
2 teaspoons reduced-salt gluten-free
    tamari

1. Place bean thread noodles in a heatproof bowl and cover with boiling water. Leave for 3–4 minutes or until noodles are soft, then drain. Rinse under running water to cool, then drain and cut noodles into short lengths (½–1 in.).

2. To make the dipping sauce, combine all ingredients in a bowl and set aside.

3. Place all the filling ingredients on a counter. Half-fill a large bowl with warm water. Dip one wrapper in the water for 10–15 seconds or until it is just soft. Drain off excess water and place on a clean surface.

4. Place a heaping teaspoon of noodles, and a few pieces each of the carrot, avocado, garlic chives, snow peas, and sprouts on the wrapper, about 1 inch in from the base of the wrapper. Fold up the bottom of the wrapper, then fold in the sides and roll up to enclose filling. Place on a tray and cover with paper towels. Continue with remaining filling and wrappers.

5. Serve the rolls on a platter with the dipping sauce.

TANGY TUNA RICE PAPER ROLLS

From The New Glucose Revolution Low GI Gluten-Free Eating Made Easy, *pages 132–136*

Per serving (per roll with dipping sauce): Calories 70 ■ Protein 5 g
Fiber 0.5 g ■ Fat 1 g (saturated fat 0.5 g) ■ Carbohydrate 9 g

GI LOW

Serves 12 ■ Preparation time: 30 minutes

2 oz. bean thread noodles

7-oz. can tuna in brine or spring water, drained

½ cup grated carrot (about 1 small carrot)

½ cup shredded Chinese cabbage

2 scallions, thinly sliced

1½ tablespoons chopped mint

¼ cup lemon juice

2 teaspoons sesame oil

1 tablespoon honey

12 round 8-inch rice papers

Dipping Sauce

⅓ cup tomato sauce

1 tablespoon reduced-salt gluten-free tamari

1. Place bean thread noodles in a heatproof bowl and cover with boiling water. Leave for 3–4 minutes or until noodles are soft, then drain. Rinse under running water to cool, drain, and then cut noodles into small lengths.

2. In a large bowl, combine tuna, carrot, cabbage, scallions, and mint, and mix well.

3. In a small bowl, whisk together the juice, oil, and honey. Pour over the tuna mixture and stir through.

4. To make the dipping sauce, combine the ingredients in a bowl. Set aside.

5. Half-fill a large bowl with warm water. Dip one wrapper in the water for 10–15 seconds or until just soft. Drain off excess water and place on a clean surface.

6. Place ¼ cup of the tuna mixture on the wrapper, about 1 inch in from the base. Fold up the bottom of the wrapper, then fold in the sides and roll up to enclose the filling. Place on a tray and cover with paper towels. Continue with remaining filling and wrappers.

7. Serve the rolls on a platter with the dipping sauce.

SALMON AND SQUASH PATTIES
WITH LIMA BEAN SALAD

To make the amount of mashed squash you need for this recipe, boil, steam, or microwave 3½ ounces peeled butternut squash. Drain off any excess liquid and mash with a fork.

From The New Glucose Revolution Low GI Gluten-Free Eating Made Easy, *page 130*

Per serving: Calories 313 ■ Protein 15 g ■ Fiber 3.5 g
Fat 24 g (saturated fat 5 g); ■ Carbohydrate 7 g

GI LOW

Serves 4 patties ■ Preparation time: 25 minutes
Chilling time: 30 minutes ■ Cooking time: 25 minutes

7-oz. can pink salmon, drained

14-oz. can lima beans, drained

⅓ cup mashed butternut squash

2 scallions, chopped

2 teaspoons rice bran

½ teaspoon gluten-free curry powder

1½ tablespoons brown rice flour

2 teaspoons canola oil

3 oz. wild arugula

Lima Bean Salad

2½ tablespoons balsamic vinegar

1½ tablespoon extra-virgin olive oil

1 small red pepper, chopped

½ small red onion, diced

1 small avocado, diced

1. In a medium bowl, mash the salmon and ½ cup lima beans with a fork. (Reserve the remaining beans for the salad.)

2. Mix in the squash, scallions, bran, and curry powder. Divide the mix into 4 portions and shape each into a patty about 3–3½ inches across. Chill in the refrigerator for 30 minutes.

3. Meanwhile, preheat the oven to 350°F. Line a baking tray with parchment paper. Dust the patties with brown rice flour. In a large frying pan, heat the canola oil, add the patties, and cook on medium heat for 1 minute each side or until just golden brown. Place the patties on a baking tray and cook in the oven for 20–25 minutes or until firm.

4. To make the Lima Bean Salad, whisk together the balsamic vinegar and oil. Combine the pepper, onion, avocado, and reserved lima beans in a small bowl. Toss with half of the balsamic dressing.

5. Place the arugula in a bowl and toss with the remaining dressing. Divide the arugula equally among four serving plates, and top each with a salmon patty and a large spoonful of lima bean salad.

TANDOORI CHICKEN WITH HERBED RICE

Per serving: Calories 420 ■ Protein 42 g ■ Fat 4.5 g (saturated fat 1 g)
Carbohydrate 51 g

GI MEDIUM

Serves 4 ■ Preparation time: 15 minutes (plus 6–8 hours for marinating)
Cooking time: 20 minutes

½ cup tandoori paste*
2 tablespoons low-fat natural yogurt,
  plus ½ cup for serving
2 tablespoons lemon juice
4 (about 4½ oz. each) boneless,
  skinless, chicken breasts
1 cup basmati rice
⅓ cup fresh coriander leaves,
  finely shredded

⅓ cup fresh mint leaves, finely shredded
rind of 1 small lime, finely grated
¼ small cucumber, finely chopped
2 ripe tomatoes, finely chopped
½ small red onion, finely chopped
pappadums, cooked following
  microwave packet instructions
⅓ cup mango chutney

1. Combine the tandoori paste, yogurt, and 1 tablespoon lemon juice in a shallow glass or ceramic dish. Use a sharp knife to make 3 slits (about ½-inch deep) in each chicken breast. Add the chicken to the tandoori mixture. Spoon the paste all over the chicken, pushing it into the slits. Cover and place in the refrigerator for 6–8 hours to marinate.

2. Preheat the oven to 400°F. Place the marinated chicken on a wire rack over a large baking dish and bake for 20 minutes, or until the chicken is no longer pink in the center and a thermometer inserted in the center of a piece registers 170°F.

3. Meanwhile, cook the rice in a large saucepan of boiling water for 10–12 minutes or until tender. Drain well and return to the pan. Set aside for 5 minutes. Add the coriander, mint, and lime rind to the rice and toss to combine.

4. Combine the extra yogurt and cucumber in a small serving bowl and mix together the tomato, onion, and remaining lemon juice in a separate bowl.

5. Serve the chicken with the herbed rice, cucumber, yogurt, tomato salsa, pappadums, and chutney.

*Available in supermarkets

LAMB BURGERS WITH SWEET POTATO CHIPS AND SPINACH SALAD

Per serving: Calories 467 ■ Protein 27 g
Fat 11 g (saturated fat 2.5 g) ■ Carbohydrate 39 g

GI LOW

Serves 6 ■ Preparation time: 20 minutes ■ Cooking time: 50 minutes

Sweet Potato Chips
2¾ lbs. sweet potato, peeled and cut
    into thick chips
1 tablespoon olive oil
salt and freshly ground black pepper,
    to taste

Lamb Burgers
1¼ lbs. ground lamb, extra lean
1 cup fresh bread crumbs, made from
    Pepperidge Farm Sprouted Wheat bread
⅓ cup fresh parsley, finely chopped
⅓ cup fresh mint, finely chopped

1 egg
1 clove garlic, crushed
½ tablespoon olive oil

Spinach Salad
4 cups baby spinach leaves
12 cherry tomatoes
1 tablespoon fresh lemon juice
freshly ground black pepper, to taste

To Serve
12-oz. jar mild tomato salsa dip

1. Preheat the oven to 425°F and line two large baking trays with nonstick baking paper.

2. To make the chips, place the sweet potato, olive oil, salt, and pepper in a large bowl and toss well to coat. Spread the sweet potato over the lined trays in a single layer. Bake for 45–50 minutes, swapping trays around once, until cooked through and crisp.

3. Meanwhile, to make the burgers, place the ground lamb, bread crumbs, parsley, mint, egg, and garlic in a large bowl. Use clean hands to mix until well combined. Divide the mixture into six portions and shape each into a round patty. Heat the olive oil in a large frying pan over medium heat. Add the patties and cook for 4–5 minutes on each side, or until the meat is no longer pink and a thermometer inserted in the center of a patty registers 160°F.

4. To make the spinach salad, combine the spinach, tomatoes, lemon juice, and pepper in a small serving bowl.

5. Serve the burgers with the sweet potato chips, salad, and salsa.

SLOW-COOKED PORK AND VEGETABLES

Per serving: Calories 360 ▪ Protein 39 g
Fat 11.5 g (saturated fat 2.5 g) ▪ Carbohydrate 18 g

GI MEDIUM

Serves 6 ▪ Preparation time: 15 minutes
Cooking time: 1 hour, 45 minutes

2½ lbs. pork neck, cut into 1½-inch pieces
2 tablespoons unbleached, all purpose flour
2 tablespoons olive oil
1 cup white wine
1½ cups chicken stock
14-oz. can diced tomatoes
8 sprigs fresh thyme
1 bunch (about 1 lb.) spring onions, chopped
3 carrots, peeled and cut into large pieces
5 medium turnips, peeled and cut into large pieces
salt and freshly ground black pepper to taste

1. Coat the pork in the flour. Heat half the oil in a large, heavy-based saucepan over medium-high heat. Add one-quarter of the pork and cook for 3–4 minutes or until well browned. Remove from the pan and repeat with the remaining pork, adding the remaining oil when necessary. Remove all the pork from the pan.

2. Increase the heat to high and add the wine to the pan. Cook, scraping any bits off the bottom of the pan, for 2–3 minutes, or until the wine is reduced by half. Return the pork to the pan with the stock, tomatoes, and thyme. Bring to the boil. Reduce the heat to low and cook, partially covered, for 30 minutes.

3. Add the spring onions, carrots, and turnips to the pan. Continue to cook, partially covered, for 1 hour, or until the vegetables and meat are very tender.

BALSAMIC LAMB WITH SWEET POTATO MASH

Per serving: Calories 370 ■ Protein 36 g
Fat 10.0 g (saturated fat 3 g) ■ Carbohydrate 33 g

GI LOW

Serves 4 ■ Preparation time: 10 minutes (plus 6 hours for marinating)
Cooking time: 20 minutes

¼ cup balsamic vinegar
2 teaspoons extra-virgin olive oil
1 clove garlic, crushed
1 tablespoon fresh rosemary leaves, chopped
4 lamb loin chops, well-trimmed (about 4¼ oz. each)
28 oz. sweet potato, peeled, cut into chunks
2 tablespoons low-fat milk*, warmed
salt and freshly ground black pepper, to taste
2 teaspoons olive oil, extra
½ cup beef stock

To Serve
7 oz. green beans, steamed
14 oz. small yellow squash, steamed

1. Combine the vinegar, extra-virgin olive oil, garlic, and rosemary
   in a shallow glass dish. Add the lamb and turn to coat. Cover and
   refrigerate for 6 hours or overnight to marinate.
2. Drain the lamb, reserving the marinade.
3. Cook the sweet potato until very tender. Drain well and mash until smooth. Add the milk and use a wooden spoon to beat until
   smooth. Season well with salt and pepper.
4. Meanwhile, heat the extra olive oil in a large frying pan over
   medium-high heat. Add the lamb and cook for 4–6 minutes on each
   side, or until a thermometer inserted in the thickest part of the
   chop registers 145°F for medium-rare or 160°F for medium well-
   done. Remove the lamb from the pan and set aside. Increase the pan
   heat to high and add the reserved marinade and the beef stock. Simmer for 2 minutes or until the sauce reduces and thickens.
5. Divide the mash among serving plates. Thickly slice the lamb and
   place over the mash. Spoon the sauce over and serve with the
   beans and squash.

   * Use low-fat soymilk if you prefer

MEDITERRANEAN CHICKEN

Per serving: Calories 582 ■ Protein 46 g
Fat 16.5 g (saturated fat 3.5 g) ■ Carbohydrate 60 g

GI LOW

Serves 4 ■ Preparation time: 10 minutes ■ Cooking time: 45 minutes

8 small chicken drumsticks
1 tablespoon olive oil
1 yellow onion, peeled
   and cut into thin wedges
2 cloves garlic, crushed
28-oz. can diced tomatoes
⅔ cup Kalamata olives

2 tablespoons tomato paste
8 oz. fusilli pasta, or other short pasta
10½ oz. broccoli, cut into small florets
⅓ cup fresh flat-leaf parsley, chopped
rind of ½ lemon, finely grated
freshly ground black pepper, to taste

1. Wrap a piece of paper towel around the end of one drumstick. Hold the paper towel with one hand and pull off the skin with the other. Discard the skin and repeat with the remaining drumsticks.

2. Heat the olive oil in a large, heavy-based saucepan over medium heat. Add half the chicken and cook for 3–4 minutes, turning occasionally until well browned. Transfer to a plate and repeat with the remaining chicken. Set aside.

3. Add the onion and garlic to the pan and cook over medium heat, stirring occasionally, for 4–5 minutes or until the onion softens. Return the chicken to the pan with the tomatoes, olives, and tomato paste. Increase the heat and bring to a boil. Reduce the heat and simmer, partially covered, for 20 minutes. Remove the lid and continue to cook for a further 5–10 minutes or until the chicken is no longer pink in the center and the sauce thickens slightly.

4. Meanwhile, cook the pasta in a large saucepan of boiling water, following the packet directions or until al dente, adding the broccoli for the last minute. Drain well and return to the pan.

5. Mix the parsley and lemon rind into the pasta. Toss well to combine and season with pepper. Serve the chicken with the broccoli pasta.

THICK VEGETABLE SOUP

The dried soup mix in this recipe is a combination of barley, red lentils, and split peas. Some brands also contain dried beans, in which case add another 15–20 minutes to the cooking time. This type of mix is available from supermarkets or health food shops. The cooled soup may be packed into airtight containers and frozen for up to three months. Freeze in single serves to make handy lunches.

Per serving: Calories 120 ■ Protein 7 g
Fat 2 g (saturated fat 0.5 g) ■ Carbohydrate 18 g

GI LOW

Serves 8 ■ Preparation time: 20 minutes ■ Cooking time: 1 hour

2 teaspoons olive oil
1 onion, chopped
2 carrots, chopped
2 celery sticks, sliced
1 cup dried soup mix
8 cups vegetable stock
14-oz. can chopped tomatoes
2 small zucchini, chopped
3 tablespoons chopped flat-leaf parsley

1. Heat the oil in a large saucepan, and add the onion, carrot, and celery. Cook over medium heat for 5 minutes, stirring occasionally, until the onion has softened.

2. Add the soup mix, stock, and tomatoes. Cover and bring to a boil, then reduce the heat to medium-low. Tilt the lid slightly, and cook for 30 minutes.

3. Add the zucchini and cook for a further 30 minutes, until all the ingredients are tender. Serve sprinkled with parsley.

Desserts and Sweet Treats

HONEY OAT BISCUITS

Per serving: Calories 98 ■ Protein 2.5 g
Fat 5 g (saturated fat 0.5 g) ■ Carbohydrate 11 g

GI MEDIUM

Makes about 24 ■ Preparation time: 10 minutes
Cooking time: 25 minutes

10 tablespoons reduced-fat margarine
½ cup 100% pure honey
1 egg
¾ cup rolled oats
1 cup almond meal
1 cup unbleached, all-purpose flour
½ teaspoon ground cinnamon

1. Preheat the oven to 350°F and line two baking trays with parchment paper.
2. Use electric beaters to beat the margarine and honey for 1 minute or until well combined. Add the egg and beat until combined. Stir in the oats and almond meal, then sift in the flour and cinnamon. Stir until well combined.
3. Shape tablespoons of the mixture into balls and place about 1 inch apart on the lined trays. Use a spoon to press down slightly. Bake for 10–12 minutes or until light and golden, swapping the trays around once in the oven during cooking. Transfer to a wire rack and repeat with any remaining mixture.

FRAGRANT RICE PUDDING WITH PLUMS

As this dessert is pretty high in carbs, it would be best served after a simple low-carb meal such as meat or fish with salad.

Per serving: Calories 296 ■ Protein 10 g
Fat 4.5 g (saturated fat 2 g) ■ Carbohydrate 52 g

GI LOW

Serves 4 ■ Preparation time: 10 minutes ■ Cooking time: 20 minutes

½ cup basmati rice
2 cups low-fat milk
1½ tablespoons granulated sugar
1 cardamom pod, lightly crushed
rind of 1 small orange, finely grated
½ teaspoon vanilla extract
½ cinnamon stick
8 plums
¼ cup pistachios, chopped, to serve

1. Cook the rice in a saucepan of boiling water for 5 minutes. Drain and return to the pan with the milk, sugar, cardamom pod, orange rind, vanilla extract, and cinnamon stick.

2. Bring to the boil, then reduce the heat to low and cook, stirring regularly, for about 15–20 minutes, until the rice is tender and creamy and the liquid is almost all absorbed. Stir constantly toward the end of the cooking time to prevent catching on the bottom.

3. Meanwhile, place the plums in a medium-sized saucepan and cover with water. Slowly bring to the boil. Reduce the heat to very low and simmer for 10 minutes. Lift the fruit from the cooking liquid with a slotted spoon, cool slightly, and slip off the skins.

4. Discard the cinnamon stick and cardamom pod from the rice, and serve immediately with the plums, sprinkled with pistachios.

CHERRY STRUDEL

Per serving: Calories 139 ▪ Protein 6 g
Fat 7 g ▪ Carbohydrate 13 g ▪ Saturated fat 2 g

GI MEDIUM

Serves 8 ▪ Preparation time: 20 minutes ▪ Cooking time: 20 minutes

8 oz. reduced-fat fresh ricotta
1 tablespoon 100% pure honey
1 teaspoon vanilla extract
1 egg, lightly beaten
5 sheets whole wheat filo pastry
olive oil spray
⅓ cup walnuts, finely chopped
8 oz. cherries, pitted

1. Preheat the oven to 375°F and line a baking tray with parchment paper.
2. Place the ricotta in a bowl and mash with a fork. Add the honey, vanilla extract, and egg, and mix until well combined.
3. Lay one filo sheet out on a work surface. Spray lightly with oil, and top with another sheet. Spray lightly with oil, and sprinkle evenly with walnuts. Top with the remaining pastry sheets, spraying lightly with oil (except for the last sheet).
4. Pile the ricotta mixture at one end of the pastry, and spread out leaving 1 inch bare pastry at each side and next to the end. The spread ricotta will be about 4 inches wide. Arrange the cherries over the ricotta.
5. Fold the end and sides over and roll up. Place on the prepared tray, seam side down. Spray lightly with oil and bake for 20 minutes, until golden brown. Allow to cool slightly before slicing to serve.

Cook's tip: Look for 100% pure honey. The commercial blends have a higher GI value.

CHOC NUT BISCOTTI

Per serving: Calories 48 ■ Protein 2 g
Fat 2.5 g (saturated fat 0.5 g) ■ Carbohydrate 5.5 g

GI MEDIUM

Makes about 50 ■ Preparation time: 30 minutes
Cooking time: 40 minutes (plus 30 minutes cooling time)

¾ cup granulated sugar

2 eggs

1 cup stone-ground whole wheat all-purpose flour

½ cup cocoa powder

⅓ cup almonds

⅓ cup pecans

⅓ cup hazelnuts

1. Preheat the oven to 350°F and line a large baking tray with parchment paper.

2. Using electric beaters, beat the sugar and eggs together for 3 minutes, until they have increased in volume and are thick and pale.

3. Sift in the flour and cocoa powder and stir with a wooden spoon until almost combined. Add the nuts, and use clean hands to mix until well combined.

4. Divide the mixture in half and shape into 2 logs about 6 inches long. Place the logs on the tray and flatten slightly to ¾-inch thick. Bake for 20 minutes, until firm. Remove from the oven and leave until completely cool.

5. Heat the oven to 250°F. Cut the logs into slices about ⅓-inch thick. Spread out onto oven trays, and bake for 20 minutes, turning once. Cool completely on wire racks. Store in an airtight container for up to one month.

PEAR AND CHOCOLATE MUFFINS

To freeze muffins, cool them completely then wrap individually in aluminum foil. Place them in a large airtight bag, and seal. Allow to thaw at room temperature for about one hour.

Per serving: Calories 203 ■ Protein 5 g
Fat 6.5 g (saturated fat 1 g) ■ Carbohydrate 32 g

GI MEDIUM

Makes 12 ■ Preparation time: 20 minutes ■ Cooking time: 20 minutes

2 cups stone-ground whole wheat self-rising flour
1 teaspoon ground cinnamon
½ cup brown sugar
1 egg
¾ cup reduced-fat milk
2 tablespoons canola oil
2 large pears, peeled and grated
¼ cup Nutella (chocolate hazelnut spread)

1. Preheat the oven to 375°F and lightly grease a 12-recess muffin tray.
2. Sift the flour and cinnamon into a large bowl and add in the husks. Add the sugar, combine, and make a well in the center.
3. Place the egg, milk, and oil in a jug or bowl and whisk with a fork until combined. Add to the dry ingredients and fold in with a large metal spoon or rubber spatula until just combined. Do not overbeat. Gently fold in the grated pear.
4. Spoon half the mixture into the bases of each muffin recess, then place 1 teaspoon of Nutella in the center of each. Top with the remaining mixture. Bake for 20 minutes, until risen, golden, and firm to a light touch. Leave in the tins for about 3 minutes, then lift out onto a wire rack to cool.

CRANBERRY AND CINNAMON POACHED PEARS WITH CUSTARD

Per serving: Calories 317 ■ Protein 7 g
Fat 4 g (saturated fat 1.5 g) ■ Carbohydrate 65 g

GI LOW

Serves 6 ■ Preparation time: 5 minutes
Cooking time: 40–50 minutes

4 cups cranberry juice
¼ cup granulated sugar
3 star anise
1 cinnamon stick, broken
6 just ripe pears, peeled

Custard
12¾-oz. can light evaporated milk
2 egg yolks
¼ cup granulated sugar
1 teaspoon vanilla extract

1. Place the cranberry juice, sugar, star anise, and cinnamon in a medium-sized saucepan (large enough to hold the pears in a single layer). Stir over low heat until the sugar dissolves. Increase the heat and bring to a simmer.

2. Add the pears to the poaching liquid. Cook, uncovered, for 40–50 minutes, turning occasionally until the pears are tender.

3. Meanwhile, to make the custard, heat the evaporated milk in another medium-sized saucepan until warmed through. Whisk the egg yolks, sugar, and vanilla together in a heatproof bowl. Whisk the warm milk into the egg yolk mixture until well combined. Pour the mixture back into the saucepan and stir over low heat for 10–15 minutes, or until the custard thickens and coats the back of a wooden spoon.

4. Serve the poached pears with a little of the syrup and the custard.

BAKED RICOTTA CHEESECAKE

Per serving: Calories 298 ■ Protein 12 g
Fat 15 g (saturated fat 6.5 g) ■ Carbohydrate 29 g

GI LOW

Serves 10 ■ Preparation time: 20 minutes
Cooking time: 1 hour, 10 minutes (plus chilling time)

Base
7 oz. oatmeal biscuits
7 tablespoons reduced-fat margarine, melted

Ricotta Filling
2½ cups reduced-fat fresh ricotta
10½ oz. silken tofu, well drained
rind of 1 lemon, finely grated
1 teaspoon vanilla extract
3 eggs
⅓ cup 100% pure honey, plus extra to serve

1. Preheat the oven to 325°F. Grease and line the base of an 8-inch (base measurement) spring form pan with parchment paper.

2. Place the biscuits in a food processor and process until fine crumbs appear. Transfer to a bowl and stir in the melted margarine. Spoon the mixture onto the base of the lined pan and use a spoon to spread evenly and press down firmly. Place in the refrigerator while you make the filling.

3. Place the ricotta, tofu, lemon rind, and vanilla in a food processor and process until smooth. Add the eggs and honey and beat until smooth and well combined. Pour the ricotta mixture over the chilled base. Bake for 1 hour to 1 hour, 10 minutes, or until the cheesecake is just set in the middle.

4. Turn the oven off and leave the cheesecake in the oven with the door slightly ajar for 1 hour to cool. Set aside at room temperature until cooled completely. Cover with plastic wrap and chill for 3–4 hours.

5. To serve, drizzle each piece of cheesecake with 1 teaspoon honey.

APPLE AND RHUBARB CRUMBLE

Per serving: Calories 306 ■ Protein 7 g
Fat 13 g (saturated fat 1.5 g) ■ Carbohydrate 33 g

GI LOW

Serves 8 ■ Preparation time: 20 minutes
Cooking time: 30–40 minutes

3 apples (such as Golden Delicious, Lady Williams, or Sundowner), peeled, cored and cut into quarters
1 bunch (about 3 cups) rhubarb, ends trimmed, washed and cut into 1½-inch lengths
2 tablespoons caster sugar

Topping
½ cup whole-grain pastry flour
1 cup almond meal
7 tablespoons reduced-fat margarine
¾ cup untoasted muesli
½ cup firmly packed brown sugar

1. Preheat the oven to 400°F and lightly grease an 8-cup ovenproof dish.

2. Layer the apples and rhubarb in the greased dish, sprinkling a little granulated sugar between layers.

3. To make the crumble topping, combine the flour and almond meal in a bowl. Use your hands to rub in the margarine until well combined and large crumbs start to form. Mix in the muesli and brown sugar.

4. Sprinkle the topping evenly over the fruit. Cover the crumble with aluminum foil and bake for 20 minutes. Remove the foil and continue to cook for a further 10–20 minutes or until the fruit is tender and the crumble golden brown. Set aside for 5 minutes before serving.

8

The Authoritative Tables of GI Values

THIS EDITION OFFERS the completely updated tables of GI values, organized alphabetically by category. These tables will help you put those low-GI food choices into your shopping cart and onto your plate. Each entry lists an individual food and its GI value, as well the nominal serving size, the amount of carbohydrate per serving, and whether the food's GI is low, medium, or high. The tables also provide each food's glycemic load (GL = [carbohydrate content x GI value] ÷ 100). We calculate the glycemic load using a "nominal" serving size as well as the carbohydrate content of that serving—both of which we've also listed. That way, you can choose foods with either a low-GI value or a low-glycemic load. If your favorite food is both high-GI and high-GL, you can either cut down the serving size or dilute the GL by combining it with very-low-GI foods, such as rice and lentils.

Key to the table

GI Value: The glycemic index value for the food, where glucose equals 100.

Nominal Serving Size: The portion of food tested.

Net Carb per Serving: The total grams of carbs available to the body for digestion from the particular food in the specific serving size (total grams of carbs minus grams of fiber).

GL per Serving: Glycemic load of the food; this relates to the quantity of carbs that will enter the bloodstream for the particular food in the specific serving size.

You can use the tables to:

- find the GI of your favorite foods
- compare carb-rich foods within a category (two types of bread or breakfast cereal, for example)
- identify the best carbohydrate choices
- improve your diet by finding a low-GI substitute for high-GI foods
- put together a low-GI meal
- find foods with a high GI but low GL

Each food appears alphabetically within a food category, such as "Bread" or "Fruit." This makes it easy to compare the kinds of foods you eat every day and helps you see which high-GI foods you can replace with low-GI versions.

The food categories are listed alphabetically, but if you need to find one quickly, check the category index below. For instance, if you wanted to find the GI value of an apple, you would look under the food category "Fruit."

The food categories used in the tables and the pages on which they begin, are:

- Beans, peas, and legumes, including baked beans, chickpeas, lentils, and split peas—page 181
- Beverages, including fruit and vegetable juices, soft drinks, flavored milk, and sports drinks—page 182
- Bread, including sliced white and whole-grain breads, fruit breads, flat breads, and crispbreads—page 185
- Breakfast cereals, including processed cereals, muesli, oats, and oatmeal—page 187

- Cakes and muffins, including other baked goods—page 189
- Cereal grains, including couscous, bulgur, and barley—page 191
- Cookies and crackers—page 191
- Dairy products, including milk, yogurt, ice cream, and dairy desserts—page 193
- Fruit, including fresh, canned, and dried fruit—page 196
- Gluten-free products—page 198
- Meals, prepared and convenience—page 200
- Meat, seafood, eggs, and protein—page 201
- Nutritional supplements—page 203
- Nuts and seeds—page 204
- Oils and dressings—page 205
- Pasta and noodles—page 205
- Rice—page 208
- Snack foods, including chocolate, fruit bars, muesli bars, nuts, and seeds—page 210
- Soups—page 215
- Soy products, including soy milk and soy yogurt—page 217
- Spreads and sweeteners, including sugars, honey, and jam—page 217
- Vegetables, including green vegetables, salad vegetables, and root vegetables—page 219

In the table, you will sometimes see these symbols:

★ indicates that a food contains little or no carbohydrate. We have included these foods—such as vegetables and protein-rich foods—because so many people ask us for their GI.

Ⓖ indicates that a food is part of the GI symbol program. Foods with the GI symbol have had their GI tested properly and are a healthy choice for their food category.

To make a fair comparison, all foods have been tested using an internationally standardized method. Gram for gram of carbohydrates, the higher the GI, the higher the blood glucose levels after consumption. If you can't find the GI value in these tables for a food you eat regularly, check our Web site (www.glycemicindex.com), where we maintain an international database of published GI values that have been tested by a reliable laboratory. Alternatively, please write to the manufacturer and encourage it to have the food tested by an accredited laboratory. In the meantime, choose a similar food from the table as a substitute.

The GI values in this book are correct at the time of publication. However, the formulation of commercial foods can change, and the GI may change as well. You can rely on foods showing the GI symbol. Although some manufacturers include the GI on the nutritional label, you would need to know that the testing was carried out independently by an accredited laboratory.

The Authoritative Tables of GI Values

Beans & Legumes

Food	GI Value	Nominal Serving Size	Available Carbs	GL Value	GI Level
Baked beans, canned in tomato sauce, Heinz	49	5 oz	18	9	low
Black beans, boiled	30	2¼ oz	15	5	low
Black-eyed beans, soaked, boiled	42	4¼ oz	17	7	low
Broad beans, frozen, reheated	63	3 oz	7	4	med
Butter beans, canned, drained	36	6 oz	17	6	low
Butter beans, dried, boiled	31	5¼ oz	17	5	low
Butter beans, soaked overnight, boiled 50 mins	26	5¼ oz	17	4	low
Cannellini beans, canned, drained	31	5 oz	14	4	low
Chickpeas, canned, drained	38	5 oz	25	10	low
Chickpeas, canned in brine	40	4 oz	16	6	low
Chickpeas, dried, boiled	28	3 oz	14	4	low
Cranberry beans, canned, drained	41	2¼ oz	17	7	low
Four-bean mix, canned, drained	37	3½ oz	14	5	low
Green beans, cooked, canned	38	2¼ oz	13	5	low
Green beans, dried, boiled	33	4 oz	15	5	low
Kidney beans, dark red, canned, drained	43	3½ oz	14	6	low
Kidney beans, red, canned, drained	36	6½ oz	19	7	low
Kidney beans, red, dried, boiled	28	3 oz	13	4	low
Kidney beans, red, soaked overnight, boiled 60 mins	51	3 oz	13	7	low

★ little or no carbs Ⓖ program participant

181

Beans & Legumes

Food	GI Value	Nominal Serving Size	Available Carbs	GL Value	GI Level
Lentils, brown, canned, drained	42	5¼ oz	21	9	low
Lentils, green, canned	48	4¾ oz	13	6	low
Lentils, green, dried, boiled	30	4½ oz	12	4	low
Lentils, red, dried, boiled	26	4½ oz	12	3	low
Lentils, red, split, boiled 25 mins	21	4½ oz	12	3	low
Lima beans, baby, frozen, reheated	32	4 oz	15	5	low
Mung beans, boiled	39	5 oz	16	6	low
Peas, dried, boiled	22	6¼ oz	13	3	low
Peas, green, frozen, boiled	48	5½ oz	13	6	low
Pinto beans, canned, drained	45	4 oz	18	8	low
President's Choice Blue Menu low-fat 4-bean salad	13	3 oz	9	1	low
Refried pinto beans, canned, Casa Fiesta	38	4 oz	20	8	low
Romano beans	46	5 oz	9	4	low
Soy beans, canned, drained	14	6 oz	5	1	low
Soy beans, dried, boiled	18	6 oz	2	0	low
Split peas, yellow, boiled 20 mins	32	6¼ oz	13	4	low
Split peas, yellow, dried, soaked overnight, boiled 55 mins	25	6¼ oz	13	3	low

Beverages

Food	GI Value	Nominal Serving Size	Available Carbs	GL Value	GI Level
All Sport Body Quencher	53	8 fl oz	16	8	low
Apple and Cherry juice, pure	43	8 fl oz	33	14	low
Apple and Mango juice, pure	47	8 fl oz	33	16	low
Apple and Pineapple juice	48	8 fl oz	34	16	low
Apple juice, filtered, pure	44	8 fl oz	30	13	low
Apple juice, Granny Smith, unsweetened	44	8 fl oz	30	13	low
Apple juice, no added sugar	40	8 fl oz	28	11	low
Apple juice with fiber	37	8 fl oz	28	10	low
Beer (4.6% alcohol)	66	25 fl oz	15	10	med
Campbell's, 100% vegetable juice	43	6 fl oz	6	3	low
Campbell's, tomato juice	33	12 fl oz	11	4	low
Campbell's V8 Splash, tropical blend fruit drink	47	8 fl oz	27	13	low
Carrot juice, freshly made	43	8 fl oz	14	6	low

★ little or no carbs   Ⓖ program participant

Beverages

Food	GI Value	Nominal Serving Size	Available Carbs	GL Value	GI Level
Chocolate Daydream shake, fructose, Revival Soy	33	8 fl oz	36	12	low
Chocolate Daydream shake, sucralose, Revival Soy	25	8 fl oz	7	2	low
Chocolate-flavored milk	37	8 fl oz	24	9	low
Chocolate milkshake, commercial	21	16 fl oz	68	14	low
Cinch Chocolate weight management powder, prepared with skim milk, Shaklee Corporation	16	8 fl oz	31	5	low
Cinch Vanilla weight management powder, prepared with skim milk, Shaklee Corporation	22	8 fl oz	29	6	low
Coca-Cola	53	12 fl oz	41	22	low
Cocoa with water	★	8 fl oz	0	0	
Coffee, black	★	8 fl oz	0	0	
Coffee, cappuccino	★	8 fl oz	4	0	
Coffee, milk	★	8 fl oz	2	0	
Cola, artificially sweetened	★	8 fl oz	0	0	
Cranberry juice cocktail	52	8 fl oz	34	18	low
Diet Coke	★	8 fl oz	0	0	
Diet dry ginger ale	★	8 fl oz	0	0	
Diet ginger beer	★	8 fl oz	0	0	
Diet lemonade	★	8 fl oz	0	0	
Diet orange fruit drink	★	12 fl oz	3	0	
Fanta orange lite	★	8 fl oz	1	0	
Fanta orange soft drink	68	8 fl oz	30	20	med
Fruit punch	67	8 fl oz	29	19	med
Gatorade	78	8 fl oz	15	12	high
Grapefruit juice, unsweetened	48	8 fl oz	18	9	low
Hot chocolate mix made with hot water	51	6 fl oz	23	12	low
Lemonade	54	8 fl oz	28	15	low
Lemonade, artificially sweetened	★	8 fl oz	0	0	
Ⓖ Lo-Gly Acai Blue	31	8 fl oz	34	11	low
Ⓖ Lo-Gly Mango Mojito	24	8 fl oz	35	8	low
Ⓖ Lo-Gly Pomegranate	28	8 fl oz	35	10	low
Ⓖ Lo-Gly Pomegranate Mojito	32	8 fl oz	31	10	low
Mango smoothie	32	8 fl oz	30	10	low
Malted powder in full-fat milk	33	8 fl oz	30	10	low
Malted powder in reduced-fat milk	36	8 fl oz	30	11	low
Malted powder in skim milk	39	8 fl oz	30	12	low
Mineral water	★	8 fl oz	0	0	

★ little or no carbs　Ⓖ program participant

Beverages

Food	GI Value	Nominal Serving Size	Available Carbs	GL Value	GI Level
MonaVie E^{MV}	52	8 fl oz	40	21	low
Nesquik powder, Chocolate, in 2% fat milk	41	8 fl oz	26	11	low
Nesquik powder, Strawberry, in 2% fat milk	35	8 fl oz	26	9	low
Orange juice, unsweetened, fresh	50	8 fl oz	19	10	low
Orange juice, unsweetened, from concentrate	53	8 fl oz	19	10	low
Pepsi Max	★	8 fl oz	0	0	
Pineapple juice, unsweetened	46	8 fl oz	24	11	low
President's Choice Blue Menu Oh Mega orange juice	48	8 fl oz	30	14	low
President's Choice Blue Menu Orange Delight Cocktail with pulp	44	8 fl oz	16	7	low
President's Choice Blue Menu Soy Beverage, Chocolate flavored	40	8 fl oz	28	11	low
President's Choice Blue Menu Soy Beverage, Original flavored	15	8 fl oz	9	1	low
President's Choice Blue Menu Soy Beverage, Vanilla flavored	28	8 fl oz	16	4	low
President's Choice Blue Menu Tomato juice, low sodium	23	8 fl oz	7	2	low
Prune juice	43	8 fl oz	36	11	low
Rice milk, low fat	86	8 fl oz	27	23	high
Slim Fast French Vanilla ready-to-drink shake	37	11 fl oz	35	13	low
Smoothie, banana	30	8 fl oz	26	8	low
Smoothie, banana and strawberry, V8 Splash	44	8 fl oz	20	9	low
Smoothie, fruit	35	8 fl oz	28	10	low
Smoothie, mango	32	8 fl oz	26	8	low
Soda water	★	8 fl oz	0	0	
Sprite Zero lemonade	★	8 fl oz	0	0	
Strawberry-flavored milk	37	8 fl oz	22	8	low
Tea, black	★	8 fl oz	0	0	
Tea, white	★	8 fl oz	1	0	
Tomato juice, no added sugar	38	8 fl oz	11	4	low
Tonic water, artificially sweetened	★	8 fl oz	0	0	
Tropical blend fruit drink	47	8 fl oz	20	9	low

★ little or no carbs   Ⓖ program participant

Bread

Food	GI Value	Nominal Serving Size	Available Carbs	GL Value	GI Level
3-grain bread, sprouted grains	55	1 oz	17	9	low
9-grain muffin	43	1 oz	11	5	low
9-grain, multigrain bread	43	1¼ oz	13	6	low
100% whole grain bread	51	1 oz	11	6	low
Apricot fruit bread	56	1½ oz	24	13	med
Bagel, white	72	1 oz	16	12	high
Baguette, traditional French bread	77	2 oz	31	24	high
Black rye bread	76	1½ oz	18	14	high
Bread roll, white	71	1 oz	17	12	high
Bread roll, whole wheat	70	1¼ oz	17	11	high
COBS Bread Higher-Fibre Low GI White Roll	50	2¼ oz	37	19	low
Continental fruit loaf	47	¾ oz	12	6	low
Corn tortilla	53	1 oz	14	7	low
Country-grain bread	61	2½ oz	28	17	med
Croissant, plain	67	1 oz	13	9	med
Crumpet	69	1¼ oz	16	11	med
Flaxseed and soy bread	55	3 oz	26	14	low
Fruit-and-spice loaf	54	2 oz	29	16	low
Gluten-free buckwheat bread	72	1 oz	11	8	high
Hamburger bun, white	61	1 oz	18	11	med
Homemade white bread	70	1¼ oz	18	13	high
Hot dog roll, white	68	1½ oz	22	15	med
Italian bread	73	1¼ oz	18	13	high
Kaiser roll, white	73	1 oz	15	11	high
Lebanese bread, white	75	1 oz	19	14	high
Light rye bread	68	1 oz	14	10	med
Melba toast, plain	70	½ oz	11	8	high
Multi-grain sandwich bread	65	1 oz	14	9	med
Natural Ovens English Muffin Bread	77	1 oz	15	12	high
Natural Ovens Happiness, cinnamon, raisin, pecan bread	63	1 oz	12	8	med
Natural Ovens Hunger Filler, whole-grain bread	59	1 oz	11	6	med
Organic stone-ground whole wheat sourdough bread	59	1¼ oz	17	10	med
Pita bread, white	63	1¼ oz	17	11	med
Pita bread, white, mini	68	1 oz	16	11	med
President's Choice Blue Menu 100% Whole Wheat Gigantico Burger Buns	62	2¾ oz	31	19	med

★ little or no carbs ⓖ program participant

Bread

Food	GI Value	Nominal Serving Size	Available Carbs	GL Value	GI Level
President's Choice Blue Menu 100% Whole Wheat Gigantico Hot Dog Rolls	62	3¼ oz	36	22	med
President's Choice Blue Menu Multi-grain Flax Loaf	51	3 oz	32	16	low
President's Choice Blue Menu Oatmeal Loaf	63	3¼ oz	43	27	med
President's Choice Blue Menu tortillas, flax	53	2 oz	29	15	low
President's Choice Blue Menu tortillas, whole wheat	59	2 oz	27	16	med
President's Choice Blue Menu Whole Grain Baguette	73	1¾ oz	21	15	high
President's Choice Blue Menu Whole Grain Chipotle Red Pepper Tortilla	35	2¼ oz	32	11	low
President's Choice Blue Menu Whole Grain Cinnamon Raisin Bagel	52	2 oz	31	16	low
President's Choice Blue Menu Whole Grain English muffins	51	2 oz	20	10	low
President's Choice Blue Menu Whole Grain Multi-Grain English Muffins	45	2 oz	20	9	low
President's Choice Blue Menu Whole Grain Multi-Grain Flax Bagel	58	2 oz	28	16	med
President's Choice Blue Menu Whole Grain Jalapeno Corn Tortilla	55	2¼ oz	32	18	low
President's Choice Blue Menu Whole Grain Oatmeal Bagel	63	2 oz	30	19	med
President's Choice Blue Menu Whole Wheat Soy Loaf	45	3 oz	27	12	low
Pumpernickel bread	50	1 oz	14	7	low
Raisin toast	63	1 oz	17	11	med
Rye bread, whole grain	58	1 oz	12	7	med
Schinkenbrot, dark rye bread	86	1¼ oz	18	15	high
Sourdough rye bread	48	1¼ oz	18	9	low
Sourdough wheat bread	54	1 oz	11	6	low
Spelt multigrain bread	54	1¼ oz	14	8	low
Stuffing, bread	74	2¾ oz	17	13	high
Traditional sourdough bread	58	3 oz	42	24	med

★ little or no carbs   Ⓖ program participant

Bread

Food	GI Value	Nominal Serving Size	Available Carbs	GL Value	GI Level
Tortilla, reduced carbohydrate	51	1 oz	7	4	low
Turkish bread, white	87	3 oz	40	35	high
White bread, high fiber, low GI	52	1¼ oz	15	8	low
White bread, regular, sliced	71	1 oz	13	9	high
White Vienna bread	66	1½ oz	23	15	med
Whole grain rye bread	58	1 oz	15	9	med
Whole wheat country grain bread	53	2½ oz	28	15	low
Whole wheat sandwich bread	71	1 oz	12	9	high
Wonder White	80	1 oz	12	10	high
Ⓖ Wonder White Low GI sandwich bread	54	1 oz	13	7	low

Breakfast Cereals

Food	GI Value	Nominal Serving Size	Available Carbs	GL Value	GI Level
All-Bran, Kellogg's	49	1 oz	23	11	low
All-Bran Complete Wheat Flakes, Kellogg's	60	1 oz	21	13	med
All-Bran Bran Buds, Kellogg's	58	1 oz	24	14	med
Bran Chex, Nabisco	58	1 oz	39	23	med
Bran Flakes, Kellogg's	74	¾ oz	14	10	high
Cheerios, General Mills	74	1 oz	21	16	high
Coco Pops, Kellogg's	80	1 oz	26	21	high
Corn Flakes, Kellogg's	86	1 oz	24	21	high
Corn Pops, Kellogg's	80	1 oz	26	21	high
Cream of Wheat	66	6 oz	29	19	med
Cream of Wheat, Instant	74	6 oz	33	24	high
Crispix, Kellogg's	87	1 oz	25	22	high
Froot Loops, Kellogg's	69	¾ oz	17	12	med
Frosted Flakes, Kellogg's	55	¾ oz	17	9	low
Gluten-free muesli	39	1½ oz	13	5	low
Golden Grahams, General Mills	71	1 oz	25	18	high
Grape-nuts, Post	71	8 oz	48	34	high
Grape-nuts Flakes, Post	80	1.1 oz	24	19	high
Hi-Bran Weet-Bix, regular	61	1 oz	17	10	med
Honey Smacks, Kellogg's	71	1 oz	23	16	high
Just Right, Kellogg's	60	1½ oz	32	19	med
Kashi 7 Whole Grain Puffs	65	0.7 oz	14	9	med
Life, Quaker Oats	66	1 oz	24	16	med

★ little or no carbs   Ⓖ program participant

Breakfast Cereals

Food	GI Value	Nominal Serving Size	Available Carbs	GL Value	GI Level
Muesli, gluten and wheat free with psyllium	50	1½ oz	13	7	low
Muesli, mixed berry & apple	64	1½ oz	30	19	med
Muesli, Natural	40	1 oz	16	6	low
Muesli, Swiss Formula	56	1 oz	18	10	med
Muesli, yeast and wheat free	44	1½ oz	13	6	low
Nutri-Grain, Kellogg's	66	¾ oz	14	9	med
Oat bran, raw, unprocessed	59	1 oz	17	10	med
Oatmeal, instant, made with water	82	6 oz	18	15	high
Oatmeal, made from steel-cut oats with water	52	6 oz	18	9	low
Oatmeal, multigrain, made with water	55	1 oz	17	9	low
Oatmeal, regular, made from oats with water	58	6 oz	18	10	med
Oats, rolled, raw	55	1 oz	15	8	low
President's Choice Blue Menu Bran Flakes	65	1 oz	24	16	med
President's Choice Blue Menu Fiber-First, multi-bran cereal	55	1 oz	23	13	low
President's Choice Blue Menu Granola Clusters, original, low-fat	63	2 oz	40	25	med
President's Choice Blue Menu Granola Clusters, Raisin Almond, low-fat	70	2 oz	40	28	high
President's Choice Blue Menu Multi-Grain Instant Oatmeal– Regular and Cinnamon & Spice	55	1½ oz	26	14	low
President's Choice Blue Menu Omega-3 Granola Cereal	43	2 oz	32	14	low
President's Choice Blue Menu Soy Crunch Multi-Grain Cereal	47	2 oz	36	17	low
President's Choice Blue Menu Steel-Cut Oats	51	1¼ oz	29	15	low
Puffed buckwheat	65	¾ oz	15	10	med
Puffed Wheat, Quaker Oats	67	1 oz	21	14	med
Quick oats	65	6 oz	19	12	med
Quick oats porridge	80	¾ oz	15	12	high
Raisin Bran, Kellogg's	61	1 oz	23	14	med
Rice Krispies, Kellogg's	82	1.2 oz	29	24	high
Semolina, cooked	87	¾ oz	17	15	high

★ little or no carbs   Ⓖ program participant

Breakfast Cereals

Food	GI Value	Nominal Serving Size	Available Carbs	GL Value	GI Level
Shredded Wheat, Post	83	1.6 oz	37	31	high
Special K, Kellogg's	69	1.1 oz	22	15	med
Total, General Mills	76	1 oz	23	17	high
Weetabix	74	1 oz	28	21	high

Cakes & Muffins

Food	GI Value	Nominal Serving Size	Available Carbs	GL Value	GI Level
9 grain muffin	43	1 oz	11	5	low
Angel food cake	67	1 oz	15	10	med
Apple, oat, raisin muffin	54	1½ oz	36	19	low
Apple berry crumble, commercially made	41	3½ oz	40	16	low
Apple muffin, homemade	46	1½ oz	17	8	low
Apricot, coconut and honey muffin	60	1½ oz	34	20	med
Banana, oat and honey muffin	65	1½ oz	17	11	med
Banana cake, homemade	51	1½ oz	17	9	low
Blueberry muffin	59	1½ oz	22	13	med
Blueberry muffin, commercially made	59	1½ oz	17	10	med
Bran muffin, commercially made	60	1½ oz	16	10	med
Carrot cake	36	1 oz	12	4	low
Carrot muffin, commercially made	62	1½ oz	17	11	med
Chocolate butterscotch muffin	53	1½ oz	31	16	low
Chocolate cake, made from packet mix with frosting, Betty Crocker	38	1 oz	14	5	low
Chocolate muffin	53	1½ oz	18	10	low
Croissant, plain	67	1 oz	13	9	med
Crumpet, white	69	1½ oz	18	12	med
Cupcake, strawberry-iced	73	1 oz	15	11	high
Double chocolate muffin	46	1½ oz	24	11	low
Doughnut, cinnamon sugar	76	1½ oz	18	14	high
Doughnut, commercially made	75	1½ oz	22	17	high
Egg custard	35	4 oz	15	5	low
Macaroons, coconut	32	1 oz	22	7	low
NutriSystem Apple Strudel Scone	43		26	11	low
NutriSystem Blueberry Bran Muffin	28	2 oz	11	3	low
NutriSystem Cranberry Orange Pastry	28	1.8 oz	19	5	low

★ little or no carbs Ⓖ program participant

Cakes & Muffins

Food	GI Value	Nominal Serving Size	Available Carbs	GL Value	GI Level
Oatmeal muffin, made from mix	69	1½ oz	17	12	med
Pancakes, buckwheat, gluten-free, packet mix	102	¾ oz	15	15	high
Pancakes, homemade	66	3 oz	20	13	med
Pancakes, prepared from mix (6-inch diameter)	67	2 oz	18	12	med
Pastry, puff	59	1 oz	15	9	med
Pound cake, Sara Lee	54	1 oz	14	8	low
President's Choice Blue Menu Cranberry & Orange Soy Muffin	48	2½ oz	29	14	low
President's Choice Blue Menu Doughnut, cake type	76	1½ oz	23	17	high
President's Choice Blue Menu Raisin Bran Flax Muffin	51	2½ oz	33	17	low
President's Choice Blue Menu Raspberry & Pomegranate Whole Grain Muffin	58	2½ oz	33	19	med
President's Choice Blue Menu Raspberry Coffee Cake	50	1¾ oz	22	11	low
President's Choice Blue Menu Whole Grain Banana & Prune Muffin	39	2½ oz	39	15	low
President's Choice Blue Menu Whole Grain Carrots, Dates, Pineapples & Walnuts Muffin	53	2½ oz	34	18	low
President's Choice Blue Menu Wild Blueberry 10-Grain Muffins	57	2½ oz	39	22	med
Scones, plain, made from packet mix	92	1 oz	17	16	high
Sponge cake, plain, unfilled	46	1 oz	14	6	low
Vanilla cake, made from packet mix with vanilla frosting, Betty Crocker	42	1½ oz	19	8	low
Waffle, plain	76	1¼ oz	16	12	high
Waffle, toasted	76	1¼ oz	16	12	high

★ little or no carbs   Ⓖ program participant

Cereal Grains

Food	GI Value	Nominal Serving Size	Available Carbs	GL Value	GI Level
Barley, pearled, boiled	25	2 oz	14	4	low
Buckwheat, boiled	54	3 oz	17	9	low
Bulgur, cracked wheat	48	3 oz	15	7	low
Millet, boiled	71	2½ oz	16	11	high
Polenta (cornmeal), boiled	68	6¾ oz	16	11	med
Quinoa, boiled	53	3½ oz	15	8	low
Rye, whole kernels	34	1 oz	14	5	low
Semolina, cooked	55	6 oz	13	7	low
Whole-wheat kernels, boiled	41	4 oz	16	7	low

Cookies & Crackers

Food	GI Value	Nominal Serving Size	Available Carbs	GL Value	GI Level
Apricot fruit cookies (97% fat free)	47	1 oz	16	8	low
Arrowroot, McCormicks's	63	¾ oz	16	10	med
Arrowroot plus, McCormicks's	62	¾ oz	16	10	med
Blueberry fruit cookies (97% fat free)	47	1 oz	16	8	low
Breton wheat crackers	67	1 oz	14	9	med
Chocolate chip cookies	43	1 oz	18	8	low
Corn Thins, puffed corn cakes, gluten-free	87	1 oz	16	14	high
Digestives, plain	62	¾ oz	15	9	med
Highland Oatcakes, Walker's	57	1 oz	13	7	med
Kavli Norwegian crispbread	71	¾ oz	14	10	high
Macaroons, coconut	32	1 oz	22	7	low
Milk Arrowroot	69	¾ oz	13	9	med
Oatmeal cookies	54	¾ oz	14	8	low
Premium Soda Crackers	74	1 oz	21	16	high
President's Choice Blue Menu Ancient Grains Snack Crackers	65	¾ oz	12	8	med
President's Choice Blue Menu Cranberry Orange Cookies	60	¾ oz	15	9	med
President's Choice Blue Menu Fat-free Fruit Bar, Apple	90	1½ oz	30	27	high
President's Choice Blue Menu Fat-free Fruit Bar, Raspberry	74	1½ oz	31	23	high
President's Choice Blue Menu Fruit Bar, Fig	70	1½ oz	30	21	high
President's Choice Blue Menu Fruit & Nut Whole Grain Soft Cookie	51	1¼ oz	24	12	low

★ little or no carbs Ⓖ program participant

Cookies & Crackers

Food	GI Value	Nominal Serving Size	Available Carbs	GL Value	GI Level
President's Choice Blue Menu Ginger and Lemon Cookies	64	¾ oz	15	10	med
President's Choice Blue Menu Oatmeal Double Chocolate Soft Cookie	49	1¼ oz	18	9	low
President's Choice Blue Menu Oatmeal Raisin Whole Grain Soft Cookie	56	1¼ oz	24	13	med
President's Choice Blue Menu Wheat and Onion Snack Crackers	60	¾ oz	14	8	med
President's Choice Blue Menu Wheat and Sesame Snack Crackers	56	¾ oz	14	8	med
President's Choice Blue Menu Wheat Snack Crackers	65	¾ oz	14	9	med
President's Choice Blue Menu Whole Wheat Fig Bar, 60%	72	1½ oz	29	21	high
Puffed crispbread	81	1 oz	18	15	high
Puffed Rice Cakes, white	82	¾ oz	15	12	high
Rice cracker, plain	91	½ oz	11	10	high
Rich tea biscuits	55	¾ oz	18	10	low
Rye crispbread	63	1 oz	28	18	med
Ryvita Fruit Crunch crispbread	66	½ oz	8	5	med
Ryvita Original Rye crispbread	69	¾ oz	10	7	med
Ⓖ Ryvita Pumpkin Seeds and Oats crispbread	48	1 oz	10	5	low
Ryvita Sesame Rye crispbread	64	¾ oz	9	8	med
Ⓖ Ryvita Sunflower Seeds and Oats crispbread	48	1 oz	9	4	low
Shortbread biscuits, plain	64	1 oz	15	10	med
Shredded Wheat cookies	62	¾ oz	15	9	med
Spicy Apple fruit cookies (97% fat free)	47	1 oz	16	8	low
Sticky Date fruit cookies (97% fat free)	47	1 oz	16	8	low
Stoned Wheat Thins	67	1 oz	19	13	med
Vanilla wafer cookies, plain	77	1 oz	16	12	high
Water cracker	63	1 oz	15	9	med
Wheat cracker, plain	70	1 oz	18	13	high
Zesty Ginger fruit cookies (97% fat free)	47	1 oz	16	8	low

★ little or no carbs   Ⓖ program participant

Dairy Products: Cheeses

Food	GI Value	Nominal Serving Size	Available Carbs	GL Value	GI Level
Brie	★	1 oz	0	0	
Camembert	★	1 oz	0	0	
Cheddar	★	1 oz	0	0	
Cheddar, 25% reduced fat	★	1 oz	0	0	
Cheddar, 50% reduced fat	★	1 oz	0	0	
Cheddar, low fat	★	1 oz	0	0	
Cheddar, reduced salt	★	1 oz	0	0	
Cheese spread, cheddar	★	1 oz	1	0	
Cheese spread, cheddar, reduced fat	★	1 oz	2	0	
Cottage cheese	★	1 oz	1	0	
Cottage cheese, low fat	★	1 oz	1	0	
Cream cheese	★	1 oz	1	0	
Cream cheese dip	★	1 oz	3	0	
Cream cheese, reduced fat	★	1 oz	1	0	
Feta	★	1 oz	0	0	
Feta, low salt	★	1 oz	0	0	
Feta, reduced fat	★	1 oz	0	0	
Mozzarella	★	1 oz	0	0	
Mozzarella, reduced fat	★	1 oz	0	0	
Parmesan	★	1 oz	0	0	
Ricotta	★	1 oz	0	0	
Ricotta, reduced fat	★	1 oz	0	0	
Soy cheese	★	1 oz	0	0	

★ little or no carbs   Ⓖ program participant

Dairy Products: Ice Cream, Custards, Puddings & Desserts

Food	GI Value	Nominal Serving Size	Available Carbs	GL Value	GI Level
Chocolate pudding, instant, made from packet with full fat milk	47	4½ oz	20	9	low
Chocolate shake, low fat chocolate soft serve with skim milk and malted milk powder	21	10 fl oz	38	8	low
Custard, homemade from milk, wheat starch and sugar	43	2 oz	14	6	low
Custard, low fat	38	4 fl oz	18	7	low
Gelato, sucrose-free, chocolate	37	2 oz	14	5	low
Gelato, sucrose-free, vanilla	39	2 oz	14	5	low
Ice cream, light creamy low fat, chocolate	27	2½ fl oz	16	4	low
Ice cream, light creamy low fat, English toffee	27	2½ fl oz	14	4	low
Ice cream, light creamy low fat, mango	30	2½ fl oz	13	4	low
Ice cream, light creamy low fat, vanilla	36	2½ fl oz	17	6	low
Ice cream, low carbohydrate, chocolate	32	3½ fl oz	5	2	low
Ice cream, regular, full fat, average	47	2½ fl oz	15	7	low
Low fat chocolate soft serve ice cream	24	2 oz	9	2	low
Low fat chocolate soft serve eaten with a plain cone	44	4 oz	20	9	low
Low fat chocolate soft serve eaten with a waffle cone	55	4 oz	28	15	low
President's Choice Blue Menu Frozen yogurt, Mochaccino	51	4 fl oz	21	11	low
President's Choice Blue Menu Frozen yogurt, Strawberry Banana	55	4 fl oz	20	11	low
President's Choice Blue Menu Frozen yogurt, Vanilla	46	4 fl oz	21	10	low
Tapioca pudding, boiled, with milk	81	4 oz	18	15	high
Vanilla frozen yogurt	46	2½ oz	17	8	low
Vanilla pudding, instant, made from packet mix with full fat milk	40	3 oz	15	6	low
Wild Berry, non-dairy, frozen fruit dessert	59	1¾ fl oz	12	7	med

★ little or no carbs   Ⓖ program participant

Dairy Products: Milk & Alternatives

Food	GI Value	Nominal Serving Size	Available Carbs	GL Value	GI Level
Blue Diamond Unsweetened Chocolate Breeze (almond beverage)	23	8 fl oz	3	1	low
Blue Diamond Unsweetened Original Breeze (almond beverage)	23	8 fl oz	2	0	low
Blue Diamond Unsweetened Vanilla Breeze (almond beverage)	23	8 fl oz	2	0	low
Chocolate-flavored, low fat milk	27	8½ fl oz	25	7	low
Chocolate-flavored milk	37	5¼ fl oz	15	6	low
Condensed milk, sweetened, full fat	61	1 oz	14	9	med
Milk, calcium-enriched, low fat (1%)	34	8 fl oz	17	6	low
Milk, low fat (1%)	32	8 fl oz	12	4	low
Milk, reduced fat (2%)	30	8 fl oz	12	4	low
Milk, whole (3.25%)	27	8 fl oz	12	3	low
Milk, with omega-3	27	8½ fl oz	16	4	low
Mocha-flavored, low fat milk	27	8½ fl oz	17	5	low
Mocha-flavored milk	32	8½ fl oz	24	8	low
Probiotic fermented milk drink with *Lactobacillus casei*	46	2¼ fl oz	12	6	low
Strawberry-flavored milk	37	6 fl oz	15	6	low
Vitasoy Light Original, soy milk	45	8 fl oz	8	4	low
Vitasoy Organic soy milk	43	8 fl oz	16	7	low
Yakult, fermented milk drink with *Lactobacillus casei*	46	2.2 fl oz	12	6	low
Yakult Light, fermented milk drink with *Lactobacillus casei*	36	2.2 fl oz	9	3	low

★ little or no carbs   Ⓖ program participant

Dairy Products: Yogurt

Food	GI Value	Nominal Serving Size	Available Carbs	GL Value	GI Level
Yogurt, low fat, natural	35	7 oz	15	5	low
Yogurt, low fat, no added sugar, vanilla or fruit	20	7 oz	17	3	low
Yoplait Original Mixed Berry yogurt	25	3½ oz	17	4	low
Yoplait Original French Vanilla yogurt	27	3½ oz	17	5	low
Yoplait Original Mango yogurt	37	3½ oz	17	6	low
Yoplait Original Strawberry yogurt	25	3½ oz	17	4	low
Yoplait Light Apple Turnover yogurt	18	7 oz	19	3	low
Yoplait Light Apricot Mango yogurt	20	7 oz	19	4	low
Yoplait Light Banana Cream Pie yogurt	18	7 oz	20	4	low
Yoplait Light Berries 'N Cream yogurt	16	7 oz	19	3	low
Yoplait Light Red Raspberry yogurt	16	7 oz	19	3	low
Yoplait Light Strawberry yogurt	16	7 oz	19	3	low

Fruit

Food	GI Value	Nominal Serving Size	Available Carbs	GL Value	GI Level
Apple	38	4 oz	13	5	low
Apple, canned, solid pack without juice	42	4½ oz	10	4	low
Apple, dried	29	1 oz	16	5	low
Apricots	57	6 oz	13	7	med
Apricots, canned, in light syrup	64	4½ oz	16	10	med
Apricots, dried	30	1 oz	16	5	low
Apricot halves, canned in fruit juice	51	4½ oz	12	6	low
Avocado	★	2¾ oz	0	0	
Banana	52	3 oz	16	8	low
Blueberries, wild	53	3½ oz	9	5	low
Breadfruit	62	2 oz	26	16	med
Cantaloupe	65	12 oz	16	10	med
Cherimoya	54	3 oz	13	7	low
Cherries, dark	63	4½ oz	15	9	med
Cherries, dried, tart	58	1½ oz	30	17	med
Cherries, frozen, tart	54	3½ oz	6	3	low
Cherries, raw, sour	22	5 oz	22	5	low
Cherries, sour, pitted, canned	41	4 oz	21	9	low
Cranberries, dried, sweetened	64	¾ oz	17	11	med

★ little or no carbs Ⓖ program participant

Fruit

Food	GI Value	Nominal Serving Size	Available Carbs	GL Value	GI Level
Dates, medjool, vacuum-packed	39	2 oz	18	7	low
Dates, pitted	45	1 oz	17	8	low
Figs	★	2 oz	8	0	
Figs, dried, tenderized	61	1 oz	16	10	med
Fruit and nut mix	15	1¼ oz	17	3	low
Fruit cocktail, canned	55	5 oz	16	9	low
Fruit salad, canned in fruit juice	54	4½ oz	15	8	low
Grapefruit	25	11 oz	15	4	low
Grapefruit, ruby red segments in juice	47	4½ oz	20	9	low
Grapes	53	3½ oz	15	8	low
Kiwi	53	6¾ oz	19	10	low
Kumquats	★	¾ oz	2	0	
Lemon	★	½ oz	0	0	
Lime	★	½ oz	0	0	
Loganberries	★	2½ oz	4	0	
Lychees, canned, in syrup, drained	79	3 oz	15	12	high
Lychees, fresh	57	2 oz	7	4	med
Mandarin segments in juice	47	4½ oz	12	6	low
Mango	51	3½ oz	13	7	low
Mixed fruit, dried	60	1 oz	18	11	med
Mixed nuts and raisins	21	1 oz	17	4	low
Mulberries	★	2½ oz	3	0	
Nectarine, fresh	43	4 oz	10	4	low
Orange	42	7 oz	15	6	low
Orange & grapefruit segments in juice	53	4½ oz	19	10	low
Papaya	56	5 oz	12	7	med
Peach	42	7 oz	13	5	low
Peach and pineapple in fruit juice	45	4½ oz	13	6	low
Peaches, canned, in heavy syrup	58	5 oz	14	8	med
Peaches, canned, in light syrup	57	4½ oz	17	10	med
Peaches, canned, in natural juice	45	5½ oz	15	7	low
Peaches, dried	35	1 oz	16	6	low
Peaches and grapes, canned in fruit juice	46	4½ oz	13	6	low
Pear	38	4 oz	16	6	low
Pear, canned, in fruit juice	43	4½ oz	14	6	low
Pear, canned, in natural juice	44	5 oz	15	7	low
Pear, dried	43	1 oz	16	7	low
Pear halves, canned, in reduced-sugar syrup, lite	25	3½ oz	15	4	low
Pineapple	59	6 oz	13	8	med

★ little or no carbs   Ⓖ program participant

Fruit

Food	GI Value	Nominal Serving Size	Available Carbs	GL Value	GI Level
Pineapple & papaya pieces, canned in juice	48	4½ oz	18	9	low
Pineapple pieces, canned in fruit juice	49	4½ oz	19	9	low
Plum	39	9 oz	19	7	low
Prunes, pitted, Sunsweet	40	1½ oz	22	9	low
Raisins	64	¾ oz	14	9	med
Raspberries	★	2 oz	3	0	
Rhubarb, stewed, unsweetened	★	3½ oz	1	0	
Strawberries	40	17 oz	13	5	low
Tropical fruit and nut mix	49	1 oz	17	8	low
Watermelon	76	10 oz	14	11	high

Gluten-free Products

Food	GI Value	Nominal Serving Size	Available Carbs	GL Value	GI Level
Apricot and Apple Fruit Strips	29	¾ oz	16	5	low
Apricot spread, no added sugar	29	1 oz	13	4	low
Buckwheat pancakes, gluten-free, packet mix	102	¾ oz	15	15	high
Cookie, chocolate-coated	35	1½ oz	18	6	low
Corn pasta	78	2 oz	15	12	high
Corn Thins, puffed corn cakes, gluten-free	87	¾ oz	16	14	high
Marmalade spread, no added sugar	27	1 oz	14	4	low
Muesli Breakfast Bar, gluten-free	50	¾ oz	13	7	low
Multigrain bread	79	1 oz	15	12	high
Pancakes, gluten-free, made from packet mix	61	3 oz	53	32	med
Pasta, rice and corn, dry	76	1 oz	19	14	high
Peach and Pear Fruit Strips	29	¾ oz	15	4	low
Plum and Apple Fruit Strips	29	1 oz	16	5	low
Raspberry spread, no added sugar	26	1 oz	14	4	low
Rice pasta, enriched (Gluten, Maize, Wheat, and Soya free)	51	¾ oz	18	9	low
Spaghetti, enriched (Gluten, Wheat, and Soya free)	51	¾ oz	19	10	low
Strawberry spread, no added sugar	29	1 oz	14	4	low

★ little or no carbs Ⓖ program participant

Meals, Prepared & Convenience

Food	GI Value	Nominal Serving Size	Available Carbs	GL Value	GI Level
Baked potato with baked beans	62	7 oz	26	16	low
Beef and ale casserole, prepared convenience meal	53	10½ oz	17	9	low
Burrito, made with corn tortilla, refried beans and tomato salsa	39	3½ oz	19	7	low
Cannelloni, spinach and ricotta, prepared convenience meal	15	8 oz	30	5	low
Chicken curry and rice, prepared convenience meal	45	10½ oz	20	9	low
Chicken fajitas	42	3 oz	6	3	low
Chicken nuggets, frozen, reheated in microwave 5 mins	46	4 oz	16	7	low
Chicken tandoori curry with rice, prepared meal	45	10 oz	53	24	low
Chow mein, chicken, prepared convenience meal	51	10½ oz	18	9	low
Creamy carbonara whole grain pasta & sauce meal	39	5 oz	21	8	low
Fish fingers	38	2½ oz	13	5	low
French fries, frozen, reheated in microwave	75	5 oz	19	14	high
French-style chicken with rice, prepared convenience meal	36	7 oz	32	12	low
Grape leaves, stuffed with rice and lamb, served with tomato sauce	30	4 oz	15	5	low
Hamburger, commercially prepared	66	3 oz	28	18	med
Lamb moussaka, prepared convenience meal	35	10½ oz	20	7	low
Lasagna, beef, commercially made	47	5 oz	17	8	low
Mashed potato, instant	85	4 oz	14	12	high
McDonald's Chicken McNuggets consumed with Sweet 'N Sour Sauce	55	4½ oz	26	14	low
McDonald's Fillet-O-Fish Burger	66	4½ oz	30	20	med
McDonald's Hamburger	66	3½ oz	25	17	med
McDonald's McChicken Burger	66	6½ oz	40	26	med
NutriSystem, Beef Stroganoff with Noodles	41	9 oz	21	9	low
NutriSystem, Cheese Tortellini	41	8 oz	25	10	low
NutriSystem, Chicken Cacciatore Parmesan	27	8 oz	16	4	low
NutriSystem, Chicken Pasta	41	9 oz	20	8	low
NutriSystem, Hearty Beef Stew	26	8 oz	16	4	low

★ little or no carbs   ⓖ program participant

Meals, Prepared & Convenience

Food	GI Value	Nominal Serving Size	Available Carbs	GL Value	GI Level
NutriSystem, Lasagna with Meat Sauce	26	8 oz	26	7	low
NutriSystem, Rotini with Meatballs	29	9 oz	25	7	low
Pizza, cheese	60	5 oz	52	31	med
Pizza, Super Supreme, pan, Pizza Hut	36	1¾ oz	14	2	low
Pizza, Super Supreme, Thin 'n Crispy, Pizza Hut	30	2½ oz	18	5	low
Pizza, Veggie Lovers, Thin 'n Crispy, Pizza Hut	49	1¾ oz	15	7	low
President's Choice Blue Menu 3-Rice Bayou Blend Rice & Beans Sidedish	44	2 oz	34	15	low
President's Choice Blue Menu 4-Rice Pilaf Rice & Beans Sidedish	46	2 oz	36	17	low
President's Choice Blue Menu 9-Vegetable Vegetarian Patty (frozen)	54	4 oz	25	14	low
President's Choice Blue Menu Barley Risotto with Herbed Chicken	38	10 oz	37	14	low
President's Choice Blue Menu Cauliflower Topped Shepherd's Pie	21	8 oz	13	3	low
President's Choice Blue Menu Deluxe Cheddar Macaroni & Cheese Dinner	34	2 oz	39	13	low
President's Choice Blue Menu Ginger Glazed Salmon	40	11 oz	45	18	low
President's Choice Blue Menu Lentil and Bean Vegetarian Patty	55	4 oz	27	15	low
President's Choice Blue Menu Linguine with Shrimp Marinara	40	11 oz	28	11	low
President's Choice Blue Menu Pasta Sauce, Tomato and Basil	33	4 oz	8	3	low
President's Choice Blue Menu Penne with Roasted Vegetable Entrée	39	11 oz	43	17	low
President's Choice Blue Menu Rice & Lentils Espana Sidedish	49	2 oz	36	18	low

★ little or no carbs   ⑤ program participant

Meals, Prepared & Convenience

Food	GI Value	Nominal Serving Size	Available Carbs	GL Value	GI Level
President's Choice Blue Menu Tricolour Linguini Sun-Dried Tomato, Basil and Original Nest	42	4 oz	57	24	low
President's Choice Blue Menu Vegetarian Chili	39	8 oz	29	11	low
President's Choice Blue Menu Whole Grain Pizza Kit	59	3¼ oz	28	17	med
Sausages	28	4 oz	9	3	low
Sausages and mashed potato, prepared convenience meal	61	10 oz	27	16	med
Shepherds' pie	66	10½ oz	22	15	med
Sirloin steak with mixed vegetables and mashed potato, homemade	66	10½ oz	25	17	med
Spaghetti bolognese, homemade	52	10½ oz	65	34	low
Stir-fried vegetables with chicken and boiled white rice, homemade	73	10½ oz	62	45	high
Sushi, salmon	48	2¾ oz	19	9	low
Taco shells, cornmeal-based, baked	68	1 oz	16	11	med

Meat, Seafood, Eggs & Protein

Food	GI Value	Nominal Serving Size	Available Carbs	GL Value	GI Level
Bacon, fried	★	1 oz	1	0	
Bacon, grilled	★	1 oz	1	0	
Beef, corned silverside	★	¾ oz	0	0	
Beef, corned silverside, canned	★	1¾ oz	0	0	
Beef, roast	★	1 oz	0	0	
Beef steak, fat trimmed	★	6 oz	0	0	
Brains, cooked	★	2 oz	0	0	
Burger, fried	★	1¾ oz	3	0	
Calamari, fried	★	2 oz	0	0	
Calamari rings, squid, not battered or crumbed	★	3 oz	2	0	
Chicken breast, baked without skin	★	3 oz	0	0	
Chicken breast, grilled without skin	★	3 oz	0	0	
Chicken chopped, cooked	★	3½ oz	0	0	
Chicken drumstick, grilled without skin	★	1½ oz	0	0	
Chicken loaf	★	¾ oz	2	0	

★ little or no carbs　 Ⓖ program participant

Meat, Seafood, Eggs & Protein

Food	GI Value	Nominal Serving Size	Available Carbs	GL Value	GI Level
Chicken roll	★	¾ oz	1	0	
Chicken thigh fillet grilled, without skin	★	1¾ oz	0	0	
Chicken wing grilled, without skin	★	¾ oz	0	0	
Cod, fried	★	4 oz	3	0	
Crab, cooked	★	2 oz	1	0	
Duck, roasted, without skin	★	2 oz	0	0	
Egg, whole, raw	★	2 fl oz	0	0	
Egg white, raw	★	1 fl oz	0	0	
Egg yolk, raw	★	½ fl oz	0	0	
Flounder, fried	★	4 oz	3	0	
Frankfurter	★	2 oz	1	0	
Ham, canned leg	★	1½ oz	0	0	
Hamburger patty	★	2¾ oz	0	0	
Kingfish (Mackerel), fried	★	4 oz	4	0	
Lamb, ground, cooked	★	3½ oz	0	0	
Lamb, grilled chop, fat trimmed	★	1¾ oz	0	0	
Lamb, roasted loin, fat trimmed	★	2 oz	0	0	
Ling (Lingcod), fried	★	4 oz	3	0	
Liver, cooked	★	2 oz	2	0	
Liverwurst	★	1 oz	0	0	
Lobster, cooked	★	2 oz	0	0	
Mullet, fried	★	4 oz	4	0	
Mussels, cooked	★	2 oz	4	0	
Nutolene	★	3 oz	4	0	
Ocean perch, fried	★	4 oz	4	0	
Octopus, cooked	★	2 oz	1	0	
Oysters, natural, plain	★	3 oz	3	0	
Pancetta	★	¾ oz	0	0	
Pepperoni	★	¾ oz	1	0	
Pork, grilled chops, fat trimmed	★	3 oz	0	0	
Prosciutto	★	1½ oz	0	0	
Quail	★	2¾ oz	0	0	
Salami	★	¾ oz	0	0	
Salmon, pink, no added salt, drained	★	2 oz	0	0	
Salmon, red, no added salt, drained	★	2 oz	0	0	
Sardines, canned in oil, drained	★	2 oz	0	0	
Sausages, fried	★	2 oz	4	0	
Scallops, cooked	★	2 oz	0	0	
Seafood marinara, canned	★	2 oz	3	0	
Shark, fried	★	4 oz	3	0	
Shrimp	★	1 oz	0	0	

★ little or no carbs   Ⓖ program participant

Meat, Seafood, Eggs & Protein

Food	GI Value	Nominal Serving Size	Available Carbs	GL Value	GI Level
Shrimp, cooked	★	2 oz	0	0	
Snapper, fried	★	4 oz	4	0	
Sole, fried	★	4 oz	3	0	
Spam, lite	★	2 oz	2	0	
Spam, regular	★	1½ oz	1	0	
Speck	★	3½ oz	0	0	
Steak, lean	★	7 oz	0	0	
Tofu, cooked	★	4½ oz	1	0	
Tofu, plain, unsweetened	★	3½ oz	0	0	
Trout, cooked	★	4 oz	0	0	
Trout, fresh or frozen	★	5¾ oz	0	0	
Trout, fried	★	4 oz	4	0	
Tuna, cooked	★	4 oz	0	0	
Tuna in brine, drained	★	2 oz	0	0	
Tuna in oil	★	2 oz	0	0	
Turkey breast, deli-sliced	★	¾ oz	0	0	
Turkey breast, rolled roast	★	3 oz	0	0	
Turkey breast, smoked, without skin	★	3 oz	0	0	
Turkey leg, roasted without skin	★	3 oz	0	0	
Turkey, roasted breast without skin	★	2¾ oz	0	0	
Veal, roasted, fat trimmed	★	3 oz	0	0	
Vegetarian sausages	★	3 oz	3	0	

Nutritional Supplements

Food	GI Value	Nominal Serving Size	Available Carbs	GL Value	GI Level
Ensure, vanilla drink	48	8 fl oz	38	18	low
Ensure Plus, vanilla	40	8 fl oz	47	19	low
Jevity, 1 cal, unflavored	48	8 fl oz	33	16	low
Jevity, 1.2 cal, unflavored	59	8 fl oz	36	21	med
Nutrimeal meal replacement drink, Usana	20	8 fl oz	17	3	low
Promote with Fiber nutritional supplement	49	8 fl oz	30	15	low
Prosure, ready-to-drink nutritional supplement, vanilla flavor	55	8 fl oz	41	23	low
TwoCal HN, high nitrogen nutritional supplement, vanilla flavor	55	8 fl oz	51	28	low

★ little or no carbs   Ⓖ program participant

Nuts & Seeds

Food	GI Value	Nominal Serving Size	Available Carbs	GL Value	GI Level
Almonds, raw	★	½ oz	1	0	
Almonds, roasted	★	½ oz	1	0	
Blue Diamond Whole Natural Almonds	25	1 oz	6	2	low
Brazil nuts	★	½ oz	0	0	
Cashew nuts, raw	22	½ oz	2	0	low
Cashew nuts, roasted and salted	22	½ oz	3	1	low
Coconut, fresh	★	½ oz	1	0	
Coconut cream	★	4 fl oz	5	0	
Coconut milk, canned	★	4 fl oz	5	0	
Coconut milk, fresh	★	4 fl oz	4	0	
Flaxseeds	★	½ oz	2	0	
Hazelnuts	★	½ oz	1	0	
Macadamia nuts, raw	★	½ oz	1	0	
Macadamia nuts, roasted	★	½ oz	1	0	
Mixed nuts, fruit, seeds	21	½ oz	4	1	low
Mixed nuts, raw	★	½ oz	1	0	
Mixed nuts, roasted, salted	24	½ oz	4	1	low
Mixed nuts, roasted, unsalted	★	½ oz	1	0	
Nut & raisin mix	★	½ oz	5	0	
Nut & seed mix	★	½ oz	1	0	
Peanut butter	★	½ oz	2	0	
Peanut butter, no added sugar	★	½ oz	1	0	
Peanuts, raw	23	1 oz	3	1	low
Peanuts, roasted	23	½ oz	3	1	low
Pecans, raw	★	½ oz	2	0	
Pine nuts	★	½ oz	1	0	
Pistachio nuts, raw	★	½ oz	2	0	
Pistachio nuts, roasted	★	½ oz	2	0	
Poppy seeds	★	¼ oz	0	0	
Pumpkin seeds, raw	★	½ oz	2	0	
Sesame seeds	★	⅓ oz	1	0	
Sunflower seeds, raw	★	½ oz	0	0	
Sunflower seeds, roasted	★	½ oz	0	0	
Walnuts	★	½ oz	0	0	

★ little or no carbs   Ⓖ program participant

Oils & Dressings

Food	GI Value	Nominal Serving Size	Available Carbs	GL Value	GI Level
Caesar salad dressing	★	1 fl oz	0	0	
Canola oil	★	⅓ fl oz	0	0	
Cream, pure, >35% fat	★	1 fl oz	1	0	
Cream, sour, >35% fat	★	1 oz	1	0	
Cream, thickened, >35% fat	★	¾ fl oz	1	0	
Dripping, pork	★	⅓ fl oz	0	0	
French dressing	★	1 fl oz	4	0	
French dressing, fat free, artificially sweetened	★	1 fl oz	0	0	
Ghee	★	⅓ oz	0	0	
Italian dressing	★	1 fl oz	2	0	
Italian dressing, fat free, artificially sweetened	★	1 fl oz	0	0	
Lard	★	⅓ oz	0	0	
Margarine, cooking	★	⅓ oz	0	0	
Mayonnaise	★	½ fl oz	3	0	
Mayonnaise, creamy, 97% fat free	★	¾ fl oz	5	0	
Salad dressing, homemade oil & vinegar	★	1 fl oz	0	0	
Safflower oil	★	⅓ fl oz	0	0	
Sesame oil	★	⅓ fl oz	0	0	
Soybean oil	★	⅓ fl oz	0	0	
Suet	★	⅓ oz	1	0	
Sunflower oil	★	⅓ fl oz	0	0	
Tartar sauce	★	1 fl oz	2	0	
Thousand Island dressing	★	¾ fl oz	4	0	
Vinegar	★	½ fl oz	0	0	

Pasta & Noodles

Food	GI Value	Nominal Serving Size	Available Carbs	GL Value	GI Level
Beef ravioli, fresh, commercially made	43	5 oz	40	17	low
Beef & vegetable ravioli, fresh, commercially made	47	5 oz	45	21	low
Cannelloni, spinach and ricotta, prepared convenience meal	15	8 oz	30	5	low
Capellini pasta, white, boiled	45	2 oz	15	7	low

★ little or no carbs　Ⓖ program participant

Pasta & Noodles

Food	GI Value	Nominal Serving Size	Available Carbs	GL Value	GI Level
Cheese & vegetable ravioli, fresh, commercially made	51	5 oz	46	23	low
Cheese tortellini, cooked	50	1¾ oz	15	8	low
Chicken & garlic ravioli, fresh, commercially made	44	5 oz	38	17	low
Corn pasta, gluten-free, boiled	78	1¾ oz	13	10	high
Couscous, boiled 5 mins	65	5½ oz	15	10	med
Creamy carbonara whole grain pasta & sauce meal	39	5 oz	21	8	low
Creamy sun-dried tomato pasta sauce	19	6 oz	15	3	low
Fettuccine, egg, fresh	54	5 oz	36	19	low
Fusilli twists, tricolor, boiled	51	2½ oz	19	10	low
Gnocchi, cooked	68	1¾ oz	15	10	med
Ⓖ Israeli Couscous, Osem brand, boiled	52	2.2 oz	20	10	low
Italian tomato & garlic pasta sauce	40	6 oz	12	5	low
Lasagna, beef, commercially made	47	5 oz	17	8	low
Lasagna sheets, fresh	49	2½ oz	22	11	low
Linguine, thick, durum wheat, boiled	46	2 oz	15	7	low
Linguine, thin, durum wheat, boiled	52	2 oz	15	8	low
Macaroni, white, durum wheat, boiled	47	2 oz	15	7	low
Macaroni and cheese, from packet mix, Kraft	64	2½ oz	19	12	med
Meat pasta sauce	24	6 oz	13	3	low
Mung bean noodles, dried, boiled	33	1¾ oz	13	4	low
Noodles, dried rice, boiled	61	2½ oz	16	10	med
Noodles, fresh rice, boiled	40	2½ oz	17	7	low
President's Choice Blue Menu 100% Whole Wheat Lasagna pasta	46	3 oz	56	26	low
President's Choice Blue Menu 100% Whole Wheat Penne Rigate pasta	51	3¼ oz	56	29	low
President's Choice Blue Menu 100% Whole Wheat Spaghetti pasta	45	3¼ oz	56	25	low
President's Choice Blue Menu 100% Whole Wheat Spaghettini	56	3¼ oz	56	31	med

★ little or no carbs   Ⓖ program participant

Pasta & Noodles

Food	GI Value	Nominal Serving Size	Available Carbs	GL Value	GI Level
President's Choice Blue Menu Fettuccini	55	4 oz	56	31	low
President's Choice Blue Menu Whole Grain Lasagna Sheets	52	2¼ oz	34	18	low
President's Choice Blue Menu Whole Wheat Rotini	57	3 oz	56	32	med
Ravioli, meat-filled, durum wheat flour, boiled	39	2 oz	13	5	low
Rice and corn pasta, gluten-free	76	2½ oz	16	12	high
Rice pasta, brown, boiled	92	5 oz	41	38	high
Rice vermicelli noodles, dried, boiled, Chinese	58	2 oz	16	9	med
Ricotta & spinach agnolotti, fresh, commercially made	47	5 oz	41	19	low
Soba noodles/buckwheat noodles	59	4 oz	24	14	med
Soba noodles, instant, served in soup	46	1¾ oz	14	6	low
Spaghetti, gluten-free, canned in tomato sauce	68	4 oz	14	10	med
Spaghetti, protein-enriched, boiled	27	1¾ oz	15	4	low
Spaghetti, white, durum wheat, boiled 10–15 mins	44	2 oz	15	7	low
Spaghetti, whole wheat, boiled	42	2 oz	15	6	low
Spaghetti with meat sauce, homemade	52	5 oz	23	12	low
Spicy tomato & bacon pasta sauce	24	6 oz	13	3	low
Spirali, white, durum wheat, boiled	43	2 oz	15	6	low
Toasted pasta, Osem brand, boiled	52	2.2 oz	20	10	low
Udon noodles, plain, boiled	62	2 oz	13	8	med
Veal tortellini, fresh, commercially made	48	5 oz	37	18	low
Vermicelli pasta, white, durum wheat, boiled	35	2 oz	15	5	low
Whole grain ricotta & spinach ravioli, fresh, commercially made	39	5 oz	37	14	low

★ little or no carbs   Ⓖ program participant

Rice

Food	GI Value	Nominal Serving Size	Available Carbs	GL Value	GI Level
Arborio risotto rice, white, boiled, SunRice	69	6.5 oz	53	37	med
Basmati rice, white, boiled	58	5.5 oz	45	26	med
Broken rice, Thai, white, cooked in rice cooker	86	6.5 oz	52	45	high
Brown Pelde rice, boiled	76	6.75 oz	46	35	high
Calrose rice, brown, medium-grain, boiled	87	6.75 oz	46	40	high
Calrose rice, white, medium-grain, boiled	83	6.5 oz	53	44	high
Doongara Clever rice, SunRice	54	5.5 oz	45	24	low
Doongara rice, brown, SunRice	66	6.75 oz	46	30	med
Glutinous rice, white, cooked in rice cooker	98	6 oz	37	36	high
Instant rice, white, cooked 6 mins with water	87	6 oz	43	37	high
Jasmine fragrant rice, SunRice	89	6 oz	48	43	high
Jasmine rice, white, long-grain, cooked in rice cooker	109	6 oz	48	52	high
Long-grain rice, white, Mahatma, boiled 15 mins	50	5.5 oz	45	23	low
Moolgiri rice	54	5.5 oz	45	24	low
Pelde parboiled rice, Sungold	87	6 oz	48	42	high
Sunbrown Quick rice, Ricegrowers, boiled	80	6.5 oz	57	46	high
SunRice Japanese-Style Sushi Rice, white	85	6 oz	47	40	high
SunRice Koshihikari rice, Ricegrowers	73	6 oz	48	35	high
SunRice Long Grain White Rice in 90 seconds, microwaved	76	4½ oz	49	37	high
SunRice Medium Grain brown rice	59	6.75 oz	46	27	med
SunRice Medium Grain Brown Rice in 90 seconds, microwaved	59	4½ oz	43	25	med
SunRice Medium Grain white rice, boiled	75	6 oz	49	37	high
SunRice Premium White Long Grain rice	59	5.5 oz	45	27	med
Uncle Ben's Converted, white, long grain, boiled 20–30 mins	50	5.5 oz	44	22	low
Uncle Ben's Original Converted, white	45	5.5 oz	44	20	low

★ little or no carbs　　Ⓖ program participant

Rice

Food	GI Value	Nominal Serving Size	Available Carbs	GL Value	GI Level
Uncle Ben's Ready Rice Long Grain & Wild (pouch)	52	5 oz	41	21	low
Uncle Ben's Ready Rice Original Long Grain (pouch)	48	5 oz	39	19	low
Uncle Ben's Ready Rice Roasted Chicken Flavored (pouch)	51	5 oz	39	20	low
Uncle Ben's Ready Rice Whole Grain Brown Rice (pouch)	48	5 oz	37	18	low
Uncle Ben's Ready Rice Whole Grain Chicken Flavored Brown Rice (pouch)	46	5¼ oz	38	17	low
Uncle Ben's Santa Fe, Ready Whole Grain Medley (pouch)	48	5.5 oz	37	18	low
Uncle Ben's Spanish Style, Ready Rice (pouch)	51	5 oz	38	19	low
Uncle Ben's Vegetable Harvest, Ready Whole Grain Medley (pouch)	48	5 oz	39	19	low
Wild rice, boiled	57	5.5 oz	35	20	med

★ little or no carbs   ⒢ program participant

Snack Foods

Food	GI Value	Nominal Serving Size	Available Carbs	GL Value	GI Level
Apricot-filled fruit bar, wholemeal pastry	50	1 oz	12	6	low
Cadbury's milk chocolate, plain	49	1 oz	16	8	low
Cashew nuts, salted	22	1¾ oz	13	3	low
Chickpea chips	44	2 oz	25	11	low
Chocolate #9 (gourmet chocolate sauce, sweetened with agave)	46	1 oz	15	7	low
Chocolate, dark, Dove	23	1 oz	23	5	low
Chocolate, dark, plain, regular	41	1 oz	15	6	low
Chocolate, milk, plain, Nestlé	42	1 oz	17	7	low
Chocolate, milk, plain, reduced sugar	35	1 oz	17	6	low
Chocolate, milk, plain, regular	41	1 oz	17	7	low
Chocolate, milk, plain, with fructose instead of regular sugar	20	1 oz	17	3	low
Chocolate brownies	42	2 oz	36	15	low
Chocolate candy, sugar free, Dove	23	1.2 oz	14	3	low
Chocolate Raspberry Zing bar, Revival Soy	47	1 bar	10	5	low
Cinch Chocolate weight management bar, Shaklee Corporation	29	1 oz	15	4	low
Cinch Lemon Cranberry weight management bar, Shaklee Corporation	23	1 oz	15	3	low
Cinch Peanut Butter weight management bar, Shaklee Corporation	22	1 oz	15	3	low
Clif bar, Chocolate Brownie Energy bar	57	2¼ oz	45	26	med
Clif Bar, Cookies 'n Cream	101	2¼ oz	42	42	high
Combos Snacks Cheddar Cheese Crackers	54	1¾ oz	30	16	low
Combos Snacks Cheddar Cheese Pretzels	52	1¾ oz	33	17	low
Corn chips	74	1 oz	17	13	high
Corn chips, plain, salted	42	1 oz	17	7	low
Dove milk chocolate	45	1 oz	17	8	low
ExtendBar Apple Cinnamon Delight Bar	33	1.35 oz	21	7	low
ExtendBar Chocolate Delight Bar	41	1.35 oz	21	9	low
ExtendBar Peanut Delight Bar	32	1.35 oz	21	7	low
Fruit and nut mix	32	2 oz	25	8	low

★ little or no carbs   Ⓖ program participant

Snack Foods

Food	GI Value	Nominal Serving Size	Available Carbs	GL Value	GI Level
Gummi confectionary, based on glucose syrup	94	¾ oz	15	14	**high**
Ironman PR bar, chocolate	39	1½ oz	19	7	**low**
Jell-O, Raspberry flavor	53	4 oz	18	10	**low**
Jelly beans	78	¾ oz	15	12	**high**
Kudos Milk Chocolate Granola Bars, Peanut Butter Flavor	45	1 oz	17	8	**low**
Kudos Milk Chocolate Granola Bars, with M&M's	52	¾ oz	16	8	**low**
Licorice, soft	78	1 oz	14	11	**high**
Life Savers, peppermint	70	½ oz	16	11	**high**
Luna Cookie Dough Bar	18	1½ oz	21	4	**low**
Luna Protein Chocolate Peanut Butter Bar	28	1½ oz	19	5	**low**
Mars Bar, regular	62	1 oz	18	11	**med**
Marshmallows, plain, pink and white	62	½ oz	15	9	**med**
Milky Bar, white, Nestlé	44	1 oz	17	7	**low**
Milky Way Bar	62	2 oz	40	25	**med**
M&M's, peanut	33	1 oz	17	6	**low**
Muesli bar, chewy, with choc chips or fruit	54	1 oz	15	8	**low**
Muesli bar, crunchy, with dried fruit	61	¾ oz	14	9	**med**
Munch Peanut Butter bar, M&M/Mars	27	1.35 oz	22	6	**low**
NutriSystem, Apple Cinnamon Soy Chips	36	1 oz	10	4	**low**
NutriSystem Apple Granola bar	52	1.4 oz	28	15	**low**
NutriSystem, Blueberry Dessert Bar	36	1½ oz	21	8	**low**
NutriSystem, Chocolate Crunch Bar	41	1 oz	15	6	**low**
NutriSystem, Chocolate	48	1½ oz	18	9	**low**
NutriSystem Cinnamon Swirl Granola bar	47	1.4 oz	27	13	**low**
NutriSystem Cranberry Granola bar	50	1.4 oz	27	14	**low**
NutriSystem Fudge Brownie	41	1.2 oz	22	9	**low**
NutriSystem Honey Mustard Pretzels	32	1 oz	7	2	**low**
NutriSystem Peanut Butter Granola bar	32	1.4 oz	18	6	**low**
Nuts, mixed, roasted and salted	24	½ oz	4	1	**low**

★ little or no carbs ⑤ program participant

Snack Foods

Food	GI Value	Nominal Serving Size	Available Carbs	GL Value	GI Level
Peanut Butter Chocolate Buddy bar, Revival Soy	52	1 bar	30	16	low
Peanuts, roasted, salted	14	5½ oz	14	2	low
Pecan nuts, raw	★	½ oz	2	0	
Performance Chocolate energy bar, Power Bar	53	2.2 oz	44	23	low
Pirate's Booty, Aged White Cheddar snack	70	1 oz	19	13	high
Pop-Tarts, double chocolate	70	1 oz	19	13	high
Popcorn, plain, cooked in microwave	72	1 oz	14	10	high
Potato chips, plain, salted	51	1¾ oz	27	14	low
PowerBar, Chocolate	53	2 oz	40	21	low
President's Choice Blue Menu 60% Whole Wheat Fig Fruit bar	72	1.35 oz	31	22	high
President's Choice Blue Menu Apple Fruit Bar, Fat-Free	90	1.35 oz	30	27	high
President's Choice Blue Menu Chewy Chocolate Chip & Marshmallow Granola Bar	78	0.9 oz	21	16	high
President's Choice Blue Menu Chewy Cranberry Apple Granola Bar	58	0.9 oz	21	12	med
President's Choice Blue Menu Fig Fruit Bar	70	1.35 oz	31	22	high
President's Choice Blue Menu Flaxseed Tortilla Chips, Sea Salt	64	1¾ oz	20	13	med
President's Choice Blue Menu Flaxseed Tortilla Chips, Spicy	64	1¾ oz	20	13	med
President's Choice Blue Menu Fruit & Nut Bar, Apple & Almonds	65	1 oz	20	13	med
President's Choice Blue Menu Fruit & Nut Mixed Berries & Almonds Chewy Multi-Grain Bars	63	1¼ oz	26	16	med
President's Choice Blue Menu Fruit & Yogurt Apple Cinnamon Chewy Bars (Soy)	34	1½ oz	21	7	low
President's Choice Blue Menu Fruit & Yogurt Cranberry Blueberry Bars (Soy)	33	1½ oz	21	7	low

★ little or no carbs   Ⓖ program participant

Snack Foods

Food	GI Value	Nominal Serving Size	Available Carbs	GL Value	GI Level
President's Choice Blue Menu Japanese Wasabi & Honey Rice & Corn Crisps	82	1¾ oz	40	33	high
President's Choice Blue Menu Microwave Popping Corn, butter flavor	72	1½ oz	31	22	high
President's Choice Blue Menu Microwave Popping Corn, natural flavor	58	1½ oz	31	18	med
President's Choice Blue Menu Original & Tomato Basil Vegetable Sticks	65	1¾ oz	38	25	med
President's Choice Blue Menu Raspberry Fruit bar, fat-free	74	1.35 oz	32	24	high
President's Choice Blue Menu Rice & Corn Chips, Japanese Tamari	91	1¾ oz	38	35	high
President's Choice Blue Menu Rice & Corn Chips, Thai Curry	84	1¾ oz	39	33	high
Pretzels, oven-baked, traditional wheat flavor	83	¾ oz	13	11	high
Rice Krispie Treat bar, Kellogg's	63	¾ oz	17	11	med
Roll-Ups, processed fruit snack	99	¾ oz	14	14	high
Skittles	70	¾ oz	18	13	high
SlimFast Meal Options bar, rich chocolate brownie flavor	64	2 oz	34	22	med
SmartZone Crunchy Chocolate Brownie Flavor Nutrition Bar	23	1.7 oz	18	4	low
SmartZone Crunchy Chocolate Caramel Flavor Nutrition Bar	16	1.7 oz	21	3	low
SmartZone Crunchy Chocolate Peanut Butter Flavor Nutrition Bar	14	1.7 oz	18	3	low
Snickers Bar	43	2 oz	34	15	low
Snickers Marathon Nutrition Bar, Dark Chocolate Crunch flavor	49	1.4 oz	15	7	low
Snickers Marathon Nutrition Bar, Honey & Toasted Almond flavor	41	1.4 oz	15	6	low
Snickers Marathon Protein Performance Bar, Caramel Nut Rush Flavor	26	2¾ oz	30	8	low

★ little or no carbs　ⓖ program participant

Snack Foods

Food	GI Value	Nominal Serving Size	Available Carbs	GL Value	GI Level
Snickers Marathon Protein Performance Bar, Chocolate Nut Burst Flavor	32	2¾ oz	26	8	**low**
SoLo GI Nutrition Bar, Berry Bliss	28	1¾ oz	22	6	**low**
SoLo GI Nutrition Bar, Chocolate Charger	28	1¾ oz	22	6	**low**
SoLo GI Nutrition Bar, Lemon Lift	28	1¾ oz	22	6	**low**
SoLo GI Nutrition Bar, Mint Mania	23	1¾ oz	22	5	**low**
SoLo GI Nutrition Bar, Peanut Power	27	1¾ oz	20	5	**low**
SoLo GI Snack Bar, Berry Bliss	28	1 oz	11	3	**low**
SoLo GI Snack Bar, Chocolate Charger	28	1 oz	10	3	**low**
SoLo GI Snack Bar, Lemon Lift	28	1 oz	11	3	**low**
SoLo GI Snack Bar, Mint Mania	23	1 oz	10	2	**low**
SoLo GI Snack Bar, Peanut Power	27	1 oz	10	3	**low**
Stretch Island Fruit Co Summer Strawberry fruit leather	29	½ oz	11	3	**low**
Twisties, cheese-flavored snack	74	1 oz	15	11	**high**
Twix bar	44	½ oz	12	5	**low**
VO2 Max Chocolate Energy Bar, M&M/Mars	49	2.2 oz	45	22	**low**
ZonePerfect nutrition bar, double chocolate flavor	44	1.7 oz	20	9	**low**

★ little or no carbs   Ⓖ program participant

Soups

Food	GI Value	Nominal Serving Size	Available Carbs	GL Value	GI Level
Black bean, canned	64	8 oz	18	12	med
Campbell's Minestrone, condensed, prepared with water	48	8 oz	28	13	low
Chicken and mushroom soup	58	8 oz	18	10	med
Clear consommé, chicken or vegetable	★	8 fl oz	2	0	
Green pea, canned	66	9 oz	19	13	med
Lentil, canned	44	9 oz	13	6	low
Minestrone, traditional	39	9 oz	13	5	low
President's Choice Blue Menu Barley Vegetable Low Fat Instant Soup	41	9 oz	28	11	low
President's Choice Blue Menu Chicken & Rotini Soup	38	9 oz	11	4	low
President's Choice Blue Menu Indian Lentil Low Fat Instant Soup	55	9 oz	20	11	low
President's Choice Blue Menu Lentil Soup	56	9 oz	19	11	med
President's Choice Blue Menu Minestrone & Pasta Instant soup, low-fat	54	9 oz	46	25	low
President's Choice Blue Menu Mushroom Barley, Ready-to-Serve	45	9 oz	9	4	low
President's Choice Blue Menu Pasta e Fagioli Soup, Ready-to-Serve	52	9 oz	22	11	low
President's Choice Blue Menu Soupreme, Carrot Soup	35	9 oz	13	5	low
President's Choice Blue Menu Soupreme, Tomato and Herb Soup	47	9 oz	14	7	low
President's Choice Blue Menu Soupreme, Winter Squash Soup	41	9 oz	10	4	low
President's Choice Blue Menu Spicy Black Bean Low Fat Instant Soup	57	9 oz	32	18	med
President's Choice Blue Menu Spicy Black Bean with Vegetables Soup	46	9 oz	34	16	low

★ little or no carbs　Ⓖ program participant

Soups

Food	GI Value	Nominal Serving Size	Available Carbs	GL Value	GI Level
President's Choice Blue Menu Spicy Thai Instant Noodles with Vegetables Low Fat Instant Soup	56	9 oz	31	17	med
President's Choice Blue Menu Vegetable CousCous Low Fat Instant Soup Cup	57	9 oz	33	19	med
President's Choice Blue Menu Vegetarian Chili, Ready-to-Serve	39	9 oz	29	11	low
President's Choice Blue Menu Vegetarian Chili Low Fat Instant Cup	36	9 oz	29	10	low
Pumpkin, Creamy, Heinz	76	7 oz	16	12	high
Split pea, canned	60	8 oz	27	16	med
Tomato, canned	45	9 oz	14	6	low
Tomato soup, condensed, prepared with water, Campbell's	52	8 oz	40	21	low
Vegetable soup	60	8 oz	18	11	med

★ little or no carbs   Ⓖ program participant

Soy Products

Food	GI Value	Nominal Serving Size	Available Carbs	GL Value	GI Level
Flaxseed and soy bread	55	3 oz	26	14	low
NutriSystem, Apple Cinnamon Soy Chips	36	1 oz	10	4	low
NutriSystem, Sour Cream and Onion Soy Chips	41	1 oz	10	4	low
President's Choice Blue Menu Soy Beverage, Chocolate flavored	40	8 fl oz	28	11	low
President's Choice Blue Menu Soy Beverage, Original flavored	15	8 fl oz	9	1	low
President's Choice Blue Menu Soy Beverage, Vanilla flavored	28	8 fl oz	16	4	low
Soy beans, canned, drained	14	6 oz	5	1	low
Soy beans, dried, boiled	18	6 oz	2	0	low
Soy yogurt, Peach and Mango, 2% fat, with sugar	50	3½ oz	8	4	low
Vitasoy Light Original, soy milk	45	12 fl oz	15	7	low
Vitasoy Organic soy milk	43	8 fl oz	16	7	low

Spreads & Sweeteners

Food	GI Value	Nominal Serving Size	Available Carbs	GL Value	GI Level
Anchovy fish paste	★	¾ oz	1	0	
Apricot 100% Pure Fruit spread, no added sugar	43	½ oz	9	4	low
Apricot fruit spread, reduced sugar	55	½ oz	6	3	low
Butter	★	⅓ oz	0	0	
Cashew spread	★	⅓ oz	3	0	
Cottee's 100% Fruit Jam Apricot	50	1 oz	15	8	low
Cottee's 100% Fruit Jam Blackberry	46	1 oz	15	7	low
Cottee's 100% Fruit Jam Breakfast Marmalade	55	1 oz	17	9	low
Cottee's 100% Fruit Jam Raspberry	46	1 oz	15	7	low
Cottee's 100% Fruit Jam Strawberry	46	1 oz	15	7	low
Dairy blend, with canola oil	★	⅓ oz	0	0	
Extra virgin olive oil spread	★	¼ oz	0	0	
Fructose, pure	19	½ oz	15	3	low

★ little or no carbs   Ⓖ program participant

Spreads & Sweeteners

Food	GI Value	Nominal Serving Size	Available Carbs	GL Value	GI Level
Ginger Marmalade, original	50	¾ oz	14	7	low
Glucose Syrup	100	¾ oz	16	16	high
Glucose tablets or powder	100	½ oz	15	15	high
Golden syrup	63	¾ oz	15	9	med
Honey, Capilano, blended	64	¾ oz	18	12	med
Honey, general	52	¾ oz	18	9	low
Honey, Ironbark	48	¾ oz	18	9	low
Honey, Red Gum	53	¾ oz	18	10	low
Honey, Salvation Jane	64	¾ oz	18	12	med
Honey, Stringybark	44	¾ oz	18	8	low
Honey, Yapunya	52	¾ oz	18	9	low
Honey, Yellow-box	35	¾ oz	18	6	low
Hummus (chickpea dip)	22	1 oz	6	1	low
Jam, sweetened with aspartame	★	⅓ oz	0	0	
Jam, sweetened with sucralose	★	⅓ oz	0	0	
Jelly, grape	52	½ oz	10	5	low
Lemon butter, homemade	★	⅓ oz	3	0	
Maple syrup, pure, Canadian	54	¾ oz	13	7	low
Margarine, canola	★	⅓ oz	0	0	
Marmalade, orange	48	½ oz	13	6	low
Marmalade, sweetened with aspartame	★	⅓ oz	0	0	
Marmalade, sweetened with sucralose	★	⅓ oz	0	0	
Nutella, hazelnut spread	33	1 oz	17	6	low
Ⓖ Premium Agave Nectar, Sweet Cactus Farms	19	¾ oz	16	3	low
President's Choice Blue Menu Twice the Fruit Apricot spread	49	½ oz	6	3	low
President's Choice Blue Menu Twice the Fruit Spread–Strawberry & Rhubarb	69	½ oz	6	4	med
Raspberry 100% Pure Fruit spread, no added sugar	26	½ oz	9	2	low
Strawberry jam, regular	51	¾ oz	13	7	low
Sugar, brown	61	½ oz	17	10	med
Sugar, white	65	½ oz	17	11	med
Tahini	★	¾ oz	0	0	

★ little or no carbs   Ⓖ program participant

Vegetables

Food	GI Value	Nominal Serving Size	Available Carbs	GL Value	GI Level
Alfalfa sprouts	★	½ oz	0	0	
Artichoke, globe	★	4 oz	2	0	
Artichoke hearts, whole, canned	★	1½ oz	1	0	
Artichokes in brine	★	1½ oz	2	0	
Artichoke hearts in brine, drained	★	3 oz	1	0	
Arugula	★	¾ oz	1	0	
Asparagus	★	3 oz	1	0	
Asparagus, canned, drained	★	3 oz	1	0	
Asparagus green/white spears, canned	★	2 oz	1	0	
Asparagus in springwater	★	2 oz	1	0	
Baby corn, cut, canned	★	1¾ oz	2	0	
Baby corn spears, whole, canned	★	1¾ oz	2	0	
Bamboo shoots, canned	★	1 oz	0	0	
Bean sprouts, cooked	★	2 oz	1	0	
Bean sprouts, raw	★	1 oz	0	0	
Beans, green	★	1¾ oz	1	0	
Beans, Chinese long	★	2½ oz	1	0	
Beets, canned	64	6 oz	16	10	**med**
Bok choy	★	3 oz	1	0	
Broccoflower	★	1½ oz	1	0	
Broccoli	★	3½ oz	1	0	
Brussels sprouts	★	2¾ oz	2	0	
Cabbage, Chinese	★	3 oz	1	0	
Cabbage, green, cooked	★	3 oz	2	0	
Cabbage, green, raw	★	3 oz	2	0	
Cabbage, red, cooked	★	3 oz	3	0	
Cabbage, red, raw	★	3 oz	3	0	
Carrots, peeled, boiled	39	3 oz	6	2	**low**
Cauliflower	★	3 oz	2	0	
Celery, cooked	★	2½ oz	2	0	
Celery, raw	★	1 oz	1	0	
Chili, banana, cooked	★	1¾ oz	1	0	
Chili, banana, raw	★	2 oz	1	0	
Chili, hot thin, cooked	★	¾ oz	1	0	
Chili, hot thin, raw	★	1 oz	1	0	
Chives	★	¼ oz	0	0	
Chayote	★	1½ oz	2	0	
Cucumber	★	1 oz	0	0	
Cucumber, Persian	★	1 oz	1	0	
Eggplant, cooked	★	1¾ oz	1	0	
Eggplant, raw	★	1½ oz	1	0	

★ little or no carbs   Ⓖ program participant

Vegetables

Food	GI Value	Nominal Serving Size	Available Carbs	GL Value	GI Level
Endive	★	3 oz	0	0	
Fennel, cooked	★	2½ oz	3	0	
Fennel, raw	★	1¾ oz	2	0	
Garlic	★	¼ oz	0	0	
Ginger	★	⅒ oz	0	0	
Green beans, sliced, canned	★	3 oz	5	0	
Green plantain, peeled, boiled, 10 mins	39	4 oz	37	14	low
Green plantain, peeled, fried in vegetable oil	40	4 oz	37	15	low
Hash browns	75	2 oz	15	11	high
Herbs, fresh or dried	★	⅒ oz	0	0	
Horseradish	★	¼ oz	1	0	
Kohlrabi	★	3 oz	4	0	
Leeks, cooked	★	3 oz	3	0	
Leeks, raw	★	3 oz	3	0	
Lettuce, Boston, Bibb	★	¾ oz	0	0	
Lettuce, cos	★	¾ oz	0	0	
Lettuce, iceberg	★	¾ oz	0	0	
Mashed potato, made with milk	85	4 oz	15	13	high
Mashed potato, made with milk and margarine	71	4.2 oz	20	14	high
Mixed vegetables, Chinese, canned	★	3 oz	5	0	
Mushrooms	★	1¼ oz	1	0	
Mushrooms, canned	★	1 oz	1	0	
Mushrooms, shiitake, canned	★	1 oz	1	0	
Okra	★	3 oz	1	0	
Onion	★	1 oz	2	0	
Onions, canned, sautéed and diced	★	1¾ oz	3	0	
Onions, sautéed and diced	★	½ oz	1	0	
Parsley, cooked	★	1½ oz	0	0	
Parsley, raw	★	¼ oz	0	0	
Parsnips, boiled	52	2¾ oz	8	4	low
Peas, green	45	7 oz	15	7	low
Pepper, green, canned	★	1½ oz	1	0	
Pepper, green, raw	★	1½ oz	1	0	
Pepper, red, canned	★	1½ oz	2	0	
Pepper, red, cooked	★	1½ oz	2	0	
Potato, baked, without skin	85	3½ oz	14	12	high
Potato, wedge, with skin	75	1¼ oz	17	13	high
Potato salad, canned	63	4 oz	16	10	med
Potato chips, deep fried	75	1½ oz	14	11	high

★ little or no carbs   Ⓖ program participant

Vegetables

Food	GI Value	Nominal Serving Size	Available Carbs	GL Value	GI Level
Potatoes, baked, Russet Burbank potatoes, baked, without fat	76	5.75 oz	41	31	high
Potatoes, boiled	59	5.75 oz	36	21	med
Potatoes, Désirée, red-skinned type, peeled, boiled 35 mins	101	4 oz	16	16	high
Potatoes, instant, mashed, Idahoan	88	4 oz	16	14	high
Potatoes, new, canned, microwaved 3 mins	65	5 oz	16	10	med
Potatoes, new, unpeeled, boiled 20 mins	78	5 oz	16	12	high
Potatoes, Ontario, white, baked in skin	60	5.75 oz	41	25	med
Potatoes, Pontiac, peeled, boiled 15 mins, mashed	91	4 oz	14	13	high
Potatoes, Pontiac, peeled, boiled whole 30–35 mins	72	4 oz	16	12	high
Potatoes, Pontiac, peeled, microwaved 7 mins	79	4 oz	16	13	high
Potatoes, red, boiled with skin on in salted water 12 mins	89	5.75 oz	37	33	high
Potatoes, red, cubed, boiled in salted water 12 mins, stored overnight in refrigerator, consumed cold	56	5.75 oz	37	21	med
Potatoes, Sebago, white, peeled, boiled 35 mins	87	4 oz	16	14	high
Pumpkin, boiled	66	7½ oz	15	10	med
Radishes, red	★	2 oz	1	0	
Rutabaga	72	5.75 oz	18	13	high
Sauerkraut, canned	★	2½ oz	1	0	
Seaweed	★	1½ oz	0	0	
Shallots, cooked	★	1 oz	1	0	
Shallots, raw	★	½ oz	1	0	
Snowpeas, cooked	★	2¾ oz	4	0	
Snowpeas, raw	★	1 oz	2	0	
Spinach, cooked	★	3 oz	1	0	
Spinach, raw	★	1 oz	0	0	
Spring onions	★	½ oz	1	0	
Squash	★	2½ oz	2	0	
Squash, butternut, boiled	51	2¾ oz	6	3	low
Sweet corn, Honey 'n Pearl variety, boiled	37	2¾ oz	15	6	low

★ little or no carbs   Ⓖ program participant

Vegetables

Food	GI Value	Nominal Serving Size	Available Carbs	GL Value	GI Level
Sweet corn, on the cob, boiled	48	2¾ oz	15	7	low
Sweet corn, whole kernel, canned, drained	46	3 oz	16	7	low
Sweet potato, baked	46	3 oz	16	7	low
Sweet potato, peeled, cubed, boiled in salted water 15 mins	59	5 oz	31	18	med
Swiss chard	★	4 oz	2	0	
Taro, boiled	54	1½ oz	15	8	low
Tomato, onion, pepper, celery	★	3 oz	3	0	
Tomato puree	★	2 oz	3	0	
Tomatoes	★	1¾ oz	1	0	
Tomatoes, in tomato juice	★	3 oz	3	0	
Tomatoes, Italian diced	★	4½ oz	5	0	
Tomatoes, Italian whole peeled Roma	★	4½ oz	5	0	
Tomatoes, whole peeled, no added salt	★	4½ oz	4	0	
Turnips	★	1¾ oz	2	0	
Water chestnuts, drained	★	¾ oz	2	0	
Watercress	★	¼ oz	0	0	
Yam, peeled, boiled	54	2½ oz	16	9	low
Zucchini, cooked	★	3 oz	2	0	
Zucchini, raw	★	2 oz	1	0	

★ little or no carbs   Ⓖ program participant

Glossary

Acanthosis nigricans: sandpaper-like dark skin located in the skin of armpits, root of the neck and, in severe cases, over joints. It is the result of severe insulin resistance. Not uncommonly, patients describe it as "dirty skin" that cannot be washed off!

Amenorrhea: when a woman has had no periods in her lifetime.

Anabolic hormone: any steroid, including synthetic preparations, which enhances constructive metabolism. They are notorious for their abuse by athletes to increase the size of their muscles.

Androstenedione: a male sex hormone weaker in activity than testosterone, produced by the ovary, testis, and adrenal glands. The body can convert it to both male and female sex steroids.

Corpus luteum: a group of cells associated with bringing the egg to maturity. It secretes the hormone progesterone in anticipation of pregnancy.

Dyslipidaemia: abnormal levels or composition of blood fats. Because these fats are water insoluble they are ferried around on proteins. These ferrying proteins specialize in the load they carry and differ in size depending on how much fat they are carrying. The "good cholesterol" is carried on a very distinct protein from the one that carries the "bad cholesterol" and those that carry triglycerides, a complex of fatty acid absorbed from food.

Fatty liver: the build-up of excessive amounts of triglycerides and other fats inside liver cells; also known as Steatohepatitis or NASH.

Follicle-stimulating hormone (FSH): a hormone produced by the pituitary gland. It affects women's ovaries, stimulating the production of an egg cell.

Glycemic load: a measure of the glycemic impact of foods based on both the type and amount of carbohydrate. It is calculated by multiplying the GI of a food by the available carbohydrate content (carbohydrate minus fiber) in a serving (expressed in grams), divided by 100.

Glycemic potential: the predicted blood glucose raising effect that a food contains.

Hirsutism: excessive growth of hair of normal or abnormal distribution. Excessive body-hair growth may be interpreted differently depending on ethnicity, complexion, and hair color. For example, relatively heavy dark body-hair growth is the rule in dark women of Mediterranean origin but may be abnormal in a blonde Swede, particularly if thick and wiry. This type of hair growth on the face, around the nipples, between the breasts, lower back, up the naval line, and inside the thighs is definitely worthy of attention.

Hypoglycemia: a condition that occurs when one's blood glucose is lower than normal, usually less than 4 mmol/L. Signs include hunger, nervousness, shakiness, perspiration, dizziness or light-headedness, sleepiness, and confusion. If left untreated, hypoglycemia may lead to unconsciousness.

Hypothalamus: a basal part of the central region of the brain that contains many regulatory centers including ones that send periodic signals to the pituitary gland, which in turn secretes specific hormones. Contrary to previous belief that the pituitary was "the master gland," with better knowledge, much of that role appears to lie with the hypothalamus.

Insulin resistance: if you are insulin resistant, your muscle and liver cells are not good at taking up glucose unless there's a lot of insulin about. Chances are you'll have very high insulin levels even long after a meal, as your body tries hard to metabolize the carbohydrate in the meal.

Luteinizing hormone (LH): a hormone produced by the pituitary gland. It plays a role in the initial production of egg cells by the ovary.

Menarche: stage of sexual development in a girl marked by the first period.

Pituitary gland: a small oval endocrine organ connected by a stalk to the hypothalamus. It is made up of two parts: the anterior (that facing forward) is involved in making and secreting several hormones, including FSH and LH.

Preeclampsia: a serious complication of late pregnancy characterized by a sudden increase in blood pressure, excessive weight gain, swelling, and protein in the urine. It requires immediate medical attention.

Sex hormones: a generic term to cover male and female sex hormones produced by testis, ovary, and adrenal gland.

Further Reading

Useful Web sites

http://www.mayoclinic.com
A reliable resource for women with PCOS in the United States. A valuable source of information regarding PCOS as well as other health conditions and links to other Web sites.

www.strongwomen.com/books
Developed by Dr. Miriam Nelson, these are written specifically for women and include easy-to-follow strength-training programs for home as well as a guide to exercises you can do at the gym.

http://www.hairfacts.com
Hair removal products tried and tested. Also links to buy products online.

http://www.diagnosemefirst.com
A comprehensive Web site covering many of the aspects of PCOS and linked conditions.

http://www.eatright.org
A good place to start looking for a dietitian near you.

http://www.pcosupport.org/
Contains valuable information on PCOS and a notice board where reader queries are addressed by other readers.

http://www.glycemicindex.com
There's a searchable GI database that's updated regularly.

http://www.gisymbol.com.au
Information about Australia's GI food labeling program.

References

Azziz, A. "The evaluation and management of hirsutism." *Obstetrics and Genecology* 101, no. 5 (2003): 995–1007.

Bradley, U., M. Spence, C. H. Courtney, M. C. McKinley, C. N. Ennis, D. R. McCance, J. McEneny, P. M. Bell, I. S. Young, and S. J. Hunter. "Low-fat versus low-carbohydrate weight reduction diets: Effects on weight loss, insulin resistance, and cardiovascular risk: A randomized control trial." *Diabetes* 58, no. 12 (2009): 2741–1248.

Brand-Miller, J. C., and S. Colagiuri. "The carnivore connection: Dietary carbohydrate in the evolution of NIDDM." *Diabetologia* 37 (1994): 1280–1286.

Carmina, E., and R. A. Lobo. "Polycystic ovary syndrome (PCOS): Arguably the most common endocrinopathy is associated with significant morbidity in women." *Journal of Clinical Endocrinology and Metabolism* 84 (1999): 1897–1899.

Corbould, A. M., S. J. Judd, and R. J. Rodgers. "Expression of types 1, 2, 3 and 3 17 beta-hyroxesteroid dehydrogenase in subcutaneous abdominal and intra-abdominal adipose tissue of women." *Journal of Clinical Endocrinology and Metabolism* 83, no. 1 (2001): 187–194.

Coviello, A. D., S. Sam, R. S. Legro, and A. Dunaif. "High prevalence of metabolic syndrome in first-degree male relatives of women with polycystic ovary syndrome is related to high rates of obesity."

The Journal of Clinical Endocrinology & Metabolism 94, no. 11 (2009): 4361–4366.

Davis, N. J., N. Tomuta, C. Schechter, C. R. Isasi, C. J. Segal-Isaacson, D. Stein, J. Zonszein, and J. Wylie-Rosett. "Comparative study of the effects of a 1-year dietary intervention of a low-carbohydrate diet versus a low-fat diet on weight and glycemic control in type 2 diabetes." *Diabetes Care* 32, no. 7 (2009): 1147–1152.

Diamond, J. "The double puzzle of diabetes." *Nature* 423, no. 6940 (2002): 599–602.

Dunaif, A. "Insulin resistance and the polycystic ovarian syndrome: Mechanisms and implications for pathogenesis." *Endocrine Reviews* 18 (1997): 774–800.

Foo, S. Y., E. R Heller, J. Wykrzykowska, C. J. Sullivan, J. J. Manning-Tobin, K. J. Moore, R. E. Gerszten, and A. Rosenzweig. "Vascular effects of a low-carbohydrate high-protein diet." *Proceedings of the National Academy of Sciences of the United States of America* 106, no. 36 (2009): 15418–15423.

Frisch, R. E. *Female fertility and the body fat connection.* University of Chicago Press: London, 2002.

Fung, T. T., R. M. van Darm, S. E. Hankinson, M. Stampfer, W. C. Willett, and F. B. Hu, "Low-carbohydrate diets and all-cause and cause-specific mortality: Two cohort studies." *Ann Intern Med* (September 7, 2010): 337–339.

Garg, A., and A. Misra. "Hepatic steatosis, insulin resistance and adipose tissue disorders." *Journal of Clinical Endocrinology and Metabolism* 87 (2002): 3019–3022.

Heraclides A., T. Chandola, D. R. Witte, and E. J. Brunner. "Psychosocial stress at work doubles the risk of type 2 diabetes in middle-aged women: Evidence from the Whitehall II study." *Diabetes Care* 32, no. 12 (2009): 2230–2235.

Jakubowicz, D. J., M. J. Iuorno, S. Jakubowicz, K. A. Roberts, and J. E. Nestler. "Effects of metformin on early pregnancy loss in polycystic ovary syndrome." *Journal of Clinical Endocrinology and Metabolism* 87 (2001): 524–529.

Kaaja, R., H. Laivuori, M. Laasko, M. J. Tikkanen, and O. Ylikorakala. "Evidence of a state of increased insulin resistance in preeclampsia." *Metabolism* 48, no. 7 (1999): 892–896.

Kirpichnikov, D., S. I. McFarklane, J. R. Sowers. "Metformin: An update." *Annals of Internal Medicine* 137, no. 1 (2002): 25–33.

Marsh, K., and J. Brand-Miller. "The optimal diet for women with polycystic ovary syndrome?" *British Journal of Nutrition* 94, no. 2 (2005): 154–165.

Marsh, K. A., K. S. Steinbeck, F. S. Atkinson, P. Petocz, and J. C. Brand-Miller. "Effect of a low glycemic index compared with a conventional healthy diet on polycystic ovary syndrome." *American Journal of Clinical Nutrition* 92, no. 1 (2010): 83–92.

Nelson, V. L., K. N. Qin, R. L. Rosenfield, J. R. Wood, T. M. Penning, R. S. Legro, J. F. Straus II, and J. M. McAllister. "The biochemical basis for increased testosterone production in theca cells propagated from patients with polycystic ovarian disease." *Journal of Clinical Endocrinology and Metabolism* 86 (2001): 5925–5923.

Ragon, N. L., R. C. Rao, S. Hwang, L. L. Alshuter, S. Elman, L. Zuckerbrow-Miller, and S. G. Korenman. "Depression in women with polycystic ovarian disease: Clinical and biochemical correlates." *Journal of Affective Disorders* 3 (2003): 299–304.

Sacks, F. M. et al. "Comparison of weight-loss diets with different compositions of fat, protein, and carbohydrates." *The New England Journal of Medicine* 360, no. 9 (2009): 859–873.

Sam, S., A. D. Coviello, Y. A. Sung, R. S. Legro, and A. Dunaif. "Metabolic phenotype in the brothers of women with polycystic ovary syndrome." *Diabetes Care* 31, no. 6 (2008): 1237–1241. Found at www.ncbi.nlm.nih.gov/pubmed/18332151.

Taubes, G. "Insulin insults may spur Alzheimer's disease." *Science* 301, no. 5629 (2003): 40–41.

Urbanek, M., R. S. Legro, D. A. Driscoll, R. Azziz, D. A. Ehrmann, R. J. Norman, J. F. Strauss, R. S. Spielman, and A. Dunaif. "Thirty-seven candidate genes for polycystic ovary syndrome: Strongest evidence for linkage is with follistatin." *Proceedings of the National Academy of Science of the United States of America* 96, no. 15 (1999): 8573–8578.

Vgontzas, A. N., R. S. Legro, A. Bixler, A. Grayerv, A. Kales, and G. P. Chrousos. "Polycystic ovarian syndrome is associated with obstructive sleep apnea and daytime sleepiness: Role of insulin resistance." *Journal of Clinical Endocrinology and Metabolism* 86 (2001): 517–520.

Yildiz, B. O., H. Yarali, H. Oguz, and M. Bayraktar. "Glucose intolerance, insulin resistance, and hyperandrogenemia in first degree relatives of women with polycystic ovary syndrome." *Journal of Clinical Endocrinology and Metabolism* 88, no. 5 (2003): 2031–2036.

Zweig, S. B., M. C. Tolentino, and L. Poretsky. "Polycystic ovarian disease." In *Principles of Diabetes Mellitus*, edited by L. Poretsky, 701–721. Kluwer Academic Publishers: Boston, 2002.

Acknowledgments

Professor Jennie Brand-Miller

I am indebted to Dr. Warren Kidson, who encouraged and inspired me to write this book. Dr. Kidson was one of the first endocrinologists in the world to recognize that women with PCOS were not only insulin resistant but that improving insulin sensitivity was the key to management.

Professor Nadir R. Farid

I am grateful to Ms. Elana Hirschowitz, who convinced me how a properly explained low-GI diet can work miracles, and Dr. Anna Louise Shankland who, despite being a young busy doctor, showed how a low-GI diet works like a dream!

Dr. Kate Marsh

My inspiration for this book came from talking to hundreds of women who struggle with PCOS and from Dr. Warren Kidson, who recognized that a low-GI diet can make a difference.

About the Authors

Jennie Brand-Miller, Ph.D., is one of the world's foremost authorities on carbohydrates and the glycemic index and has championed the GI approach to nutrition for more than twenty-five years. Professor of Nutrition at the University of Sydney and past president of the Nutrition Society of Australia, Brand-Miller directs a GI food-labeling program in Australia (www.gisymbol.com.au) with Diabetes Australia and the Juvenile Diabetes Research Foundation to ensure that claims about the GI are scientifically correct and are applied only to nutritious foods. Winner of Australia's prestigious ATSE Clunies Ross Award in 2003 for her commitment to advancing science and technology, Brand-Miller is always in demand as a speaker, and her laboratory at the University of Sydney is recognized worldwide for research on carbohydrates and health.

Professor Nadir R. Farid began his academic career at the Memorial University of Newfoundland, Canada. He became Professor of Medicine and Endocrinology in 1984 and of Cell Sciences in 1989. An internationally recognized investigative and clinical endocrinologist, he trained many scientists, internists, and endocrinologists, and described or redefined a number of clinical syndromes. Dr. Farid has edited five books and published in excess of 450 scientific papers, reviews, and chapters. He was founder and CEO of Osancor Biotech, Inc. and was a consultant at 119 Harley Street and The Wellington Hospital, both in London, England. Dr. Farid passed away in early 2010.

Dr. Kate Marsh is an Advanced Accredited Practicing Dietitian and Credentialed Diabetes Educator, with a Masters of Nutrition and Dietetics from the University of Sydney (1995) and a Graduate Certificate in Diabetes Education and Management from the University of Technology, Sydney (1997). She has recently completed her Ph.D. at the University of Sydney, looking at the benefits of a low-GI diet in the management of insulin resistance in women with PCOS and has published a number of scientific papers. Kate works in private practice in Sydney, Australia and has a particular interest in PCOS, having worked with hundreds of women with this condition over the past few years. She chairs a PCOS interest group for dietitians, frequently speaks to both dietitians and women with PCOS on the dietary management of this condition, and is a member of the PCOS Alliance, which is currently working on developing best practice guidelines for the management of PCOS in Australia. Kate is also coauthor of *The Low GI Vegetarian Cookbook, Low GI Gluten-Free Living* and *PCOS Made Easy* (an audio CD program), contributed the dietary chapter for a textbook on PCOS, and writes regularly for a number of magazines on diabetes, PCOS, insulin resistance, and vegetarian nutrition.

Index

Recipe Index